7-MINUTE
BODY
PLAN

LUCY WYNDHAM-READ

CONTENTS

7-MINUTE
BODY
PLAN

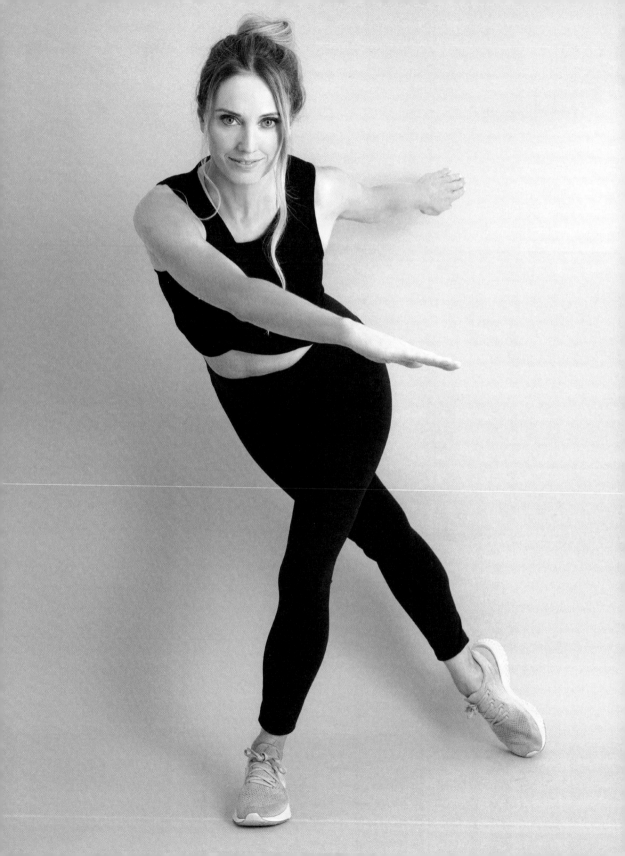

THE RECIPES

THE 7-MINUTE BODY PLAN FOR LIFE

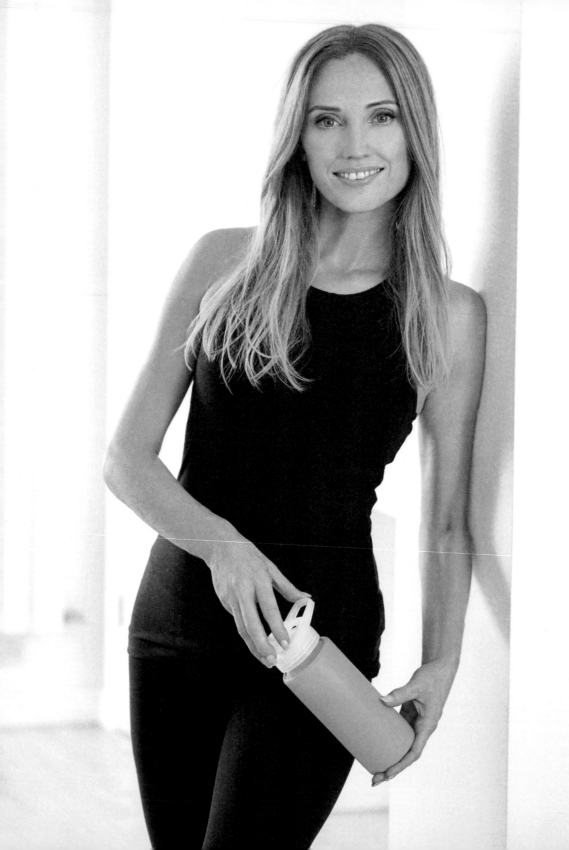

INTRODUCTION

Whether you're big, small, use a wheelchair, are young, old, fit, or just starting out on your fitness journey, this book is for you. It gives you 7 different workouts, each only 7 minutes long and containing 7 different exercises, every one of which is designed to get you maximum results. Every workout also has 7 tips to go with it, to help you to get the most out of those 7 days. Plus there are loads of quick, easy, and healthy recipes, to take you from breakfast through lunch and dinner, with snacking and smoothies to help you along the way.

This book will give you all the information you need to look fabulous and feel amazing, both inside and out, in only 7 minutes a day. Owning this book is just like having a life-long gym membership at home, because all the workouts are home-based, and you don't need to invest in any equipment, because each move uses your own body weight to get you in tip-top shape.

The whole book is peppered with my advice on the easy way to lead – and maintain – a healthy lifestyle. By the end of the book, you will have a new ability to tailor your very own 7-exercises-in-7-minutes workout, with 49 highly effective moves to choose from.

And the book finishes up by handing over to you, giving you 7 tips for motivation and maintenance, after the workouts have given you the power to take control of your own health, your body, and your mind.

Before we start, I want to tell you how I know that my 7-minute workouts will work for you. I'll explain to you my passion, my mission, and why I am super-excited to work alongside you now, to help you look and feel your best.

Let's go back to the beginning. This often really surprises my clients, but it's true: I dreaded sports and fitness at school. I gave every excuse in the book to get out of any lesson that required physical activity all through my school years, both because of bullying and because I had zero confidence. Yet deep down I knew I was desperate to be a strong and confident girl, not one to hide away or be walked over.

So after finishing school I knew I had to do something drastic. So I made what was, for me, the most unlikely move: I joined the Army. To say it shocked my parents is an understatement. But I knew I would never be able to ask the Sergeant Major if I could get out of sports!

I had jumped out of my comfort zone and straight into the deep end.

I remember so clearly arriving at the barracks, aged 19, and thinking to myself: what have I done? But it proved to be one of the best decisions I've ever made. It made me realize I could do anything I put my mind to, as fitness became a part of my daily routine. I was able to run! I could do everything that I didn't think I could at school. Very quickly, I started to fall in love with fitness, which in turn helped boost my confidence and self-esteem. The more I challenged myself, the more I grew as a person.

I spent five years in the Army, then threw myself into studying to become a personal trainer. I will always remember my first day working at a local private health club. The gym manager showed me around and explained that they had more than 1,800 members. I was shocked, as the gym space was so tiny, so I quickly counted how many treadmills, bikes, steppers, and rowing machines there were. The total came to 20 – just 5 of each – so I asked the obvious question: "What happens if all 1,800 members turn up at the same time?" He laughed and confidently said, "That won't happen. Only 11 per cent of members ever use the gym!"

To him that was a great success, as it meant a big fat profit, but to me it was terribly saddening. The other 89 per cent of members had paid to improve their health and wellbeing, but something was stopping them from going to the gym. It was at that moment that I made it my mission to help that 89 per cent to get fit at home and discover what they are truly capable of, and how to be their best, just as I had discovered by joining the Army.

I worked in that gym for 4 weeks, then quickly set up my own personal training service, offering fitness training at home. An ad in the local paper delivered more than 40 enquiries in a single day, and I have never looked back.

I am all about making fitness accessible and – let's be honest – nothing is more accessible than your front room. I have helped literally hundreds of thousands of people of all abilities, ages, and sizes become their best. You can meet some of them on pp.14–17.

I have poured 25 years of experience – and my heart and soul – into giving you a book to simply make you look and feel your best, and I am so excited to be on this journey with you.

Lucy xx

Lucy xx
(your trainer and biggest believer)

THE 7-MINUTE WORKOUT THAT WENT VIRAL

In late January 2018, I sat at home uploading a 7-minute Lose Belly Fat video to my YouTube channel. Little did I know that it was to become one of the most-liked workout videos on YouTube and that – in over a year – it would reach 44 million views (and still going strong). But one thing that did not surprise me was the feedback from viewers, saying, "I can't believe this works!" Well, of course, I knew it would, which is why I created it.

Traditional workouts focus on isolated moves, such as the plank, or a bicep curl, or a wall-seated holding squat. But even though these are working set muscles, they are not engaging many, nor are they putting the body through its fullest range of motion, so those workouts will not achieve the full calorie-burning effect.

I use a special combination of cardio-toning moves and multicompound and multidirectional exercises (see p10). This means you are engaging hundreds of muscles in one move. Throughout the 7-minute workouts in this book, we work all 3 planes of motion that your body travels through, to get the maximum calorie burn. As a trainer, I am all about getting results for my clients, so every move of my 7-minute workouts achieves the maximum effect.

Plus, you do each of the 7 moves for 60 seconds, so we are also working on endurance. It is at the 40-second mark when any exercise in this book begins to feel challenging. And, as in life, it is only when you challenge yourself that you get results. It is in those last 20 seconds that the magic happens, and, as it is only 20 seconds, you can keep going, as the end is in sight!

But even better than that, my specially created moves achieve a great calorie burn. They help to induce an effect known as EPOC (Excess Post Oxygen Consumption), so you naturally increase your calorie burn for hours after the workout has finished. This is simply because your body is still working hard to rebalance its hormones, restock its fuel stores, cool down, and return to its normal state. EPOC is epic...

The last great bonus of my workouts is – of course – that they are short! That makes them do-able. Everyone can find 7 minutes within their day. You can too, trust me. You just need to prioritize your own wellbeing.

My workouts have helped millions of people worldwide to get in shape and boost their health, and have proved you can feel your best in just 7 minutes a day.

7 REASONS WHY

MY WORKOUTS WORK

1 DO-ABLE.
They are quick. To be precise, each workout is just 7 minutes long, so they are easy to squeeze in first thing in the morning, or at any time in the day, unlike longer workouts.

2 FUN.
Each 7-minute workout has 7 different moves, so you never get bored and you are not repeating moves for long. The time will fly by.

3 HIGHER CALORIE BURN.
Each of the 49 moves in this book focuses on what I call MCM and MDM (Multicompound Moves and Multidirectional Moves). In a nutshell, this means each move is working for a maximum calorie burn, and will be toning hundreds of muscles. The more toned your body is, the more calories it will burn every day.

4 INTENSITY, NOT DURATION.
I cannot stress this enough: intensity is more effective than duration. Many people feel that the longer they spend working out, the more effective it will be. Actually it is more important to focus on pushing yourself to your maximum. Let's compare two of my clients' stories here.

Example 1

Taylor is at the gym on the treadmill, lightly jogging, for 45 minutes. She can't run super-fast, as she wouldn't be able to for more than 20–40 seconds. She burns off calories, but it takes a long time (more than an hour, when you add the time to get to the gym and back). And she'll have paid a pretty sum for that gym membership. Yet she could get a better result in a shorter time at home for free.

Example 2

Susie lives a super-busy life, and so keeps in tip-top shape by doing 7-minute workouts at home. Each of the 60-second cardio-tone moves takes her intensity up higher than Taylor's, so Susie burns more calories. The key to shorter workouts is that you can push yourself. And you don't need to be a fitness fan: anyone can do them, a beginner, someone who is feeling overweight, or who has a disability.

5 KEEP IT SIMPLE.

These 7-minute workouts are super-simple to follow, unlike other plans. And because you know exactly what you are doing, it gives you the confidence to keep going and put in 100 per cent. This is where my KISMIE (Keep It Simple, Make It Easy) rule jumps in. Clarity is what we need with a fitness regime; anything complicated will confuse us.

6 NO EQUIPMENT NEEDED.

In all my 7-minute workouts, we focus on using your own body weight, so you don't need any equipment. Bodyweight training is a super-effective way to strengthen, sculpt, and tone your body. Bodyweight exercises also make it easy to move quickly from one move to the next, meaning you need shorter rest times, so you keep that intensity up, you are working harder, and – again – are burning more calories. You also get to improve your flexibility. Bodyweight exercises win, hands down.

7 WORK OUT ANYWHERE.

All my 7-minute workouts can be done in the smallest of spaces. You don't need to put your healthy lifestyle on hold if you are travelling. Just pack this book in your luggage and get fit wherever you are. Consistency is key and it is also what will bring those amazing results, plus these workouts will soon become part of your life and you won't want to stop.

WHY 7 DAYS?

I have found that people are more likely to stick to my 7-day plan, because nearly everyone can commit to just a week of working out. Often, if you offer someone a 90-day plan, for instance, it can seem never-ending and impossible to commit to, and so – well – they don't last the entire time.

The beauty of the 7 workouts in this book is that you won't get bored. After your first 7 days, simply pick another workout for the next week. And nothing is more motivational than to kick off a new week with a new goal to achieve. Every Monday, I see a huge spike online for views of my 7-minute workout videos.

You have structure, you have confidence, and you know what you are doing. See? KISMIE! Keep It Simple, Make It Easy.

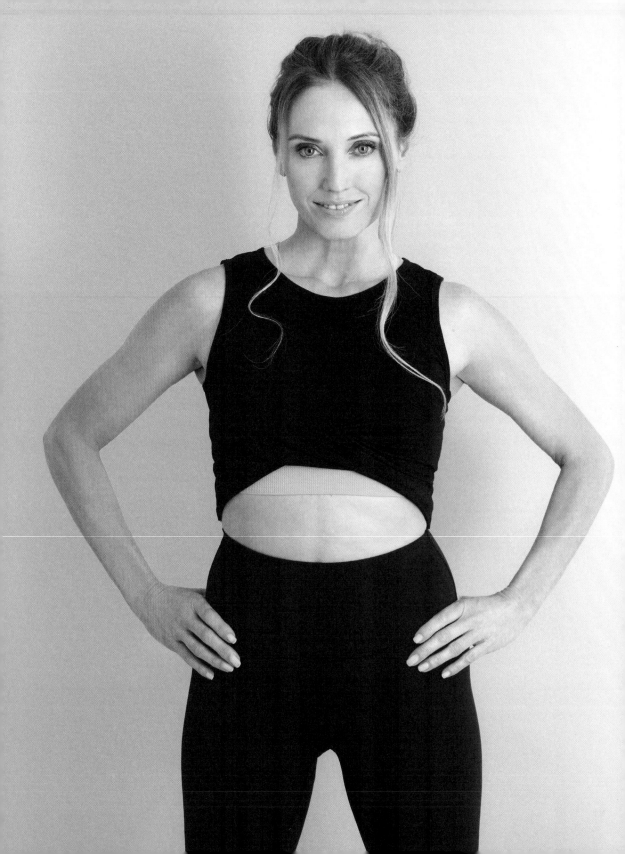

AMAZING RESULTS

I can confidently say that if you stick to my 7-minute 7-day challenges,ß alongside healthy eating and the right mindset, you will see and feel results.

We are all unique, and we all see results at different rates. In the book I have shared with you some incredible before-and-after success stories (see p14–17); they are here to inspire you, but not to compare yourself to, and you will see how all their results have varied.

Working out for 7 minutes is incredible for your health, and this – if I am honest – is what excites me more than the visible inch loss, because your inner health is the most valuable thing you have.

So, just remember that results come not just from what you see on the outside, but also from what is happening on the inside, and your mental wellbeing. No matter what, every time you work out, *this* is what you will be doing:

You will be...

√ burning off excess body fat
√ improving your health
√ increasing your energy levels
√ strengthening your bones
√ losing inches

√ increasing your fitness levels
√ boosting your confidence
√ improving circulation
√ increasing your flexibility
√ improving your co-ordination
√ improving your posture
√ enhancing your natural calorie-burn
√ reducing anxiety
√ able to sleep better
√ improving your heart health
√ investing time in you
√ buzzing with that feel-good factor
√ building a natural inclination to make healthier food choices
√ sculpting up all over
√ strengthening your immune system
√ noticing your glowing skin

And that's just a few of the benefits – the list goes on and on...

7-MINUTE BODY PLAN

SUCCESS STORIES

*Around the world, people have been getting into Lucy's 7-minute workouts,
with incredible results. Here are just a handful of their inspirational stories.*

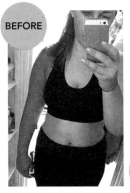
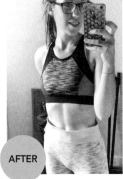

BEFORE

AFTER

Beth Collins, 22

FROM HAMPSHIRE, UK
E-COMMERCE MARKETING EXECUTIVE

"I have been following Lucy's workouts for more than
3 years now and, for the last 18 months, I've been at
my ideal weight. I just had a very indulgent birthday,
but I am confident I'll get back on track.
   "I love how easy the workouts are to follow and
they really have changed my life."

BEST RESULT
I've always been self-conscious about my legs and
I really see a difference. They look slim and toned.

FAVOURITE WORKOUTS
Melt off belly fat; Love my legs (see p32 and p68)

IN LUCY'S SQUAD
3 years

RESULTS
Lost 32kg (70lb / 5 stone)

Amy Dunford, 33

FROM MANITOBA, CANADA
MOTHER OF 2, PART-TIME HOSPITAL ADMINISTRATOR

"I decided to do Lucy's 7-minute belly fat workout, as,
though I'm at my ideal weight, I had extra weight on
my belly. After losing that, her workouts helped me
tone the extra skin.
   "I didn't expect to see a difference, but I lost 5cm
(2in) from my waist in a week! It makes me want to eat
better, keep moving, and be the best version of me."

BEST RESULT
Showing my kids a healthy lifestyle and a happy mom.

FAVOURITE WORKOUTS
Melt off belly fat (see p32)

IN LUCY'S SQUAD
1 year

RESULTS
Lost 45kg (99lb / 7 stone 1lb)

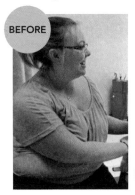
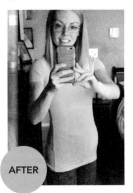

BEFORE

AFTER

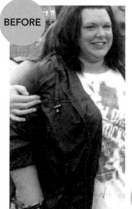
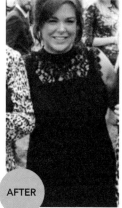

BEFORE

AFTER

Victoria Sutcliffe, 33

FROM EAST YORKSHIRE, UK
PURCHASE LEDGER CLERK

"I have come a long way. I've already lost 32kg (70lb / 5 stone) and am aiming to lose 6kg (13lb / 1 stone) more. I love these workouts as I can do them at home, they are free, and they are easy to fit into a busy day. Most days I try and do at least 2, plus a power walk if I can, but I have found that even if I do just 1 every day it makes a difference.

"I have PCOS and I am due to start IVF this year, on the proviso that I lose weight. Lucy's workouts are the only thing that has helped me, as well as keeping my nutrition in check. So as well as the amazing fact I will soon be able to start IVF, I certainly have more energy and confidence.

"My muscle tone has really impressed me too, and it gets better every week. I am able to wear clothes – and even jewellery – that I couldn't before."

BEST RESULT

My top result is muscle tone. I love seeing definition in my arms and legs getting better and better.

FAVOURITE WORKOUTS

Dream arms (see p50)

IN LUCY'S SQUAD

18 months

RESULTS

Lost 32kg (70lb / 5 stone)

Claire Jones, 45

FROM SURREY, UK
ENTREPRENEUR AND COMPANY DIRECTOR

"I broke my foot 5 years ago and have since had operations and procedures to try and fix it, but with no success. I had to give up running, which had a huge impact on my fitness and weight.

"Having listened to Lucy talk about the workouts, I decided it was time to give them a go. I've dropped 2 dress sizes, reduced my blood pressure to a normal level, and have a body weight in the optimum range for the first time in more than a decade.

"The 7-minute workouts are all you have to do on a daily basis. They work every muscle, increase your fitness levels, and tone your whole body. They're easy to fit in and you get results in 7 days. When I was told my foot was permanently broken, I never thought I'd find another exercise to fill the gap. But I am addicted to 7-minute workouts; they're a big part of my life."

BEST RESULT

Finally being comfortable in my body and loving how I look for the first time in well over a decade.

FAVOURITE WORKOUTS

Dream arms; Love my legs; Seated cardio-boost & sculpt; Calorie-burning (see p50, p68, p86, p104)

IN LUCY'S SQUAD

9 months

RESULTS

Lost 12.7kg (28lb / 2 stone) and 31cm (12.5in) over her body

BEFORE

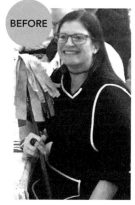
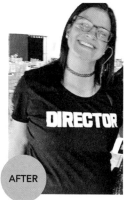

AFTER

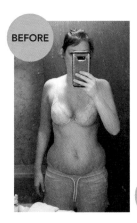

BEFORE

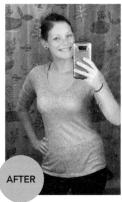

AFTER

Amber Amis, 26

FROM PENNSYLVANIA, USA
MOTHER OF 3, PART-TIME STUDENT NURSE

"I found Lucy's workouts 6 months before I started them, to get a better grip on my mental health and learn to take control of the little things. I am so glad I took the chance! The first time I did a 7-minute challenge, yes, by minute 3 I thought I was dying, I was so out of shape, but I pushed through. I only gave myself weekly goals (because I usually quit), but, by week 3, I had the confidence to do her workouts twice a day. I was in shock that I could do it!

"My mood is better, I am able to keep up with my kids, and I actually feel like me again, which hasn't happened in a long while. I have even managed to encourage some friends and family to join me on this amazing journey together, not only of weight loss, but a journey of better self-help mentally. Thank you so much Lucy for giving me the courage and strength to know that I can do it."

BEST RESULT

My mental attitude has improved by 110%. I have more energy to handle my 3 young children and way more confidence in myself.

FAVOURITE WORKOUTS

Melt off belly fat (see p32)

IN LUCY'S SQUAD

9 months

RESULTS

Lost 8kg (18lb / 1 stone 4lb)

Sue Beech, 43

FROM WEST MIDLANDS, UK
SPECIAL EDUCATIONAL NEEDS TEACHING ASSISTANT

"I began Lucy's exercising routine about 18 months ago. I was concerned about the risk of diabetes and so adjusted my diet, reducing the carbs and sugar I was eating and increasing my vegetable and water intake. I didn't believe I'd ever lose the weight, so I didn't begin with a weight goal in mind. What spurred me on was wanting better confidence, better sleep, more energy, and less water retention. Once I was into the routine, I found my co-ordination and balance also improved.

"I do like to mix it up and I follow 2 workouts 4 times a week, targeting various areas. As former military, I missed the routine of exercising, as it is so important for morale. I enjoy the wellbeing I have gained and, as a busy working mother, I love doing something for me. Thanks for everything."

BEST RESULT

My new-found confidence has led me to university, to study supporting children.

FAVOURITE WORKOUTS

Melt off belly fat workout; Dream arms (see p32, p50)

IN LUCY'S SQUAD

18 months

RESULTS

Lost more than 12.7kg (28lb / 2 stone)

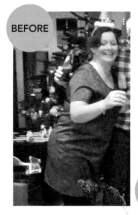

BEFORE

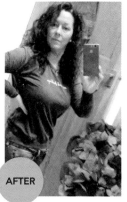

AFTER

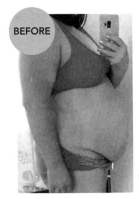

BEFORE

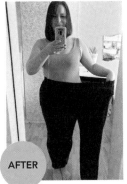

AFTER

Kelly Wood, 40

FROM BEDFORDSHIRE, UK
MOTHER OF 5

"My New Year's resolution was to lose weight… To be honest this has been my New Year's resolution for 20 years and, by January 31, it's usually over. But this year I came across Lucy's 7-minute workouts. I thought I'd give it a go, and to my astonishment, by the end of 7 days, I had lost 6cm (2½in) from my waist. And the bonus was that I had enjoyed doing the workout each day, and actually wanted to do more.

"I have tried home workouts before, but got bored after 10 minutes. I only had to find 7 minutes to do Lucy's workouts, so it was so much more do-able. I look forward to working out in the morning. I am fitter, healthier, and stronger than I have ever been. I haven't just lost weight, my whole figure has changed.

"I'm a mother of 5 and never get a lot of sleep, but as soon as I have done my workout I feel energized and ready for anything. It's changed my life."

BEST RESULT

With each week I feel myself becoming stronger and fitter, and my confidence grows and grows.

FAVOURITE WORKOUTS

Melt off belly fat workout (see p32)

IN LUCY'S SQUAD

10 months

RESULTS

Lost 15kg (33lb / 2 stone 5lb); 18cm (7in) from my waist; 10cm (4in) from each arm; 15cm (6in) from my hips; 8cm (3in) from each thigh

Morgan Goudy, 32

FROM UTAH, USA
MOTHER OF 4

"I have 3 boys, 1 daughter, 2 dogs, 2 cats, and 1 bearded dragon. I have been obese most of my adult life. I gained weight with every pregnancy and thought of working out as a punishment and avoided it as much as I could. Now I need it! It helps my mental health just as much as my physical health.

"I started doing Lucy's legs workout every day. After a month, I started doing 2 workouts a day. After 2 months I started doing 3 a day, and then worked my way up to doing an hour at a time.

"Lucy's workouts have changed my life. They have helped me reach my goals and helped me overcome obstacles in my life. She has taught me how to be consistent, and that hard work does pay off.

"I was diagnosed in March with spondylolisthesis, which is a slipped vertebrae. Lucy's standing ab workouts have helped so much with my back pain."

BEST RESULT

Lucy has taught me a positive and "can-do" attitude.

FAVOURITE WORKOUTS

Love my legs; Little black dress (see p68, p122)

IN LUCY'S SQUAD

10 months

RESULTS

Lost 32kg (70lb / 5 stone), 20cm (8in) from my waist, 18cm (7in) from my bust and behind, and 13cm (5in) around my thighs

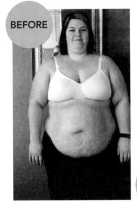

BEFORE

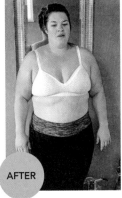

AFTER

HOW TO
USE THIS BOOK

In this book you will find 7 different 7-minute workouts to follow. You simply complete a 7-minute routine once a day for 7 days. In each case, I will describe how to measure your progress, then break down each of the moves, including all my tips on how to perform the exercise safely, correctly, and effectively.

So each week you pick a new routine. At the beginning of each workout, I have suggested how you can measure yourself to see the best results for that challenge. I've also given 7 tips for how to boost your results during that week, and added some FAQs that I hear all the time, relevant to each workout.

SCHEDULE YOUR WORKOUT

I recommend that you aim to work out in the morning, so you can get it done early in the day. Sometimes, if you leave it until later on in the day, other things – such as social life, or family matters – can get in the way. But don't worry if life interferes from time to time; as each workout is only 7 minutes long, you're pretty likely to find that time before bed. So if you're not a morning person, fear not: your results will be the same whatever time you work out.

Better still, you can even start creating your own 7-minute workouts. If you flip to p30, you will see how to divide the exercises in different ways, to suit your lifestyle, whether you are sitting down all day, or on your feet, are recovering from an injury, or are a new mother, or going through the menopause. I wanted to create these to help you to tailor your own workout to your own life stage and lifestyle.

MEASURE YOUR INTENSITY

Intensity is key to getting results, and I have a useful scale that means you can be sure

All 7 workouts will help boost your calorie burn, tone you up, increase your energy, and – of course – make you feel utterly fabulous.

that you are working out to the right intensity to get your desired results. As with any exercise, you get out what you put in. You want to be feeling slightly out of breath, but not to a point of utter exhaustion; equally don't let it be too easy. Hitting the right intensity is what gives you incredible results.

Score yourself on a scale of 1–10 for your perceived rate of exertion:

1 Not exhausted at all (as if you are seated)

2 Very, very light (as if you are walking around at home)

3 Very light gentle exercise

4 Moderate (easily able to hold a conversation)

5 Somewhat hard (feeling a little out of breath)

6 Feeling challenged and out of breath, so it would be hard to hold a full conversation

7 Very hard (not able to talk)

8 Very, very hard

9 Near exhaustion

10 Maximal

To get the best results, you should aim to be in the 5–6 zone, as this is the fat-burning zone.

WHAT YOU NEED

This section is going to be short, as you really don't need much. In fact, only 3 things!

First, you need a timer or a clock with a clearly visible second hand, as all the exercises in this book are performed for 60 seconds. Most smartphones have stopwatches, and there are lots of free apps offering timers that bleep you through a countdown of the last few seconds.

Second is clothing. Don't worry, you don't need to rush out and buy lots of new fitness gear, but I do recommend a good-quality sports bra and a good pair of training shoes. That's it. And, because you are working out at home, you can throw on any old pair of leggings, or a ropey old holey T-shirt.

Oh, yes, there is one more thing you'll need: dedication. No matter what, focus on sticking to the workout plan for 7 days. It will be *so* worth it.

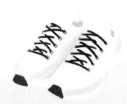

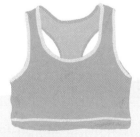

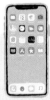

TRAINING SHOES
You don't need to spend a fortune, just make sure that your shoes fit and have good stability.

SPORTS BRA
It's worth finding a robust and well-fitting one; avoid yoga bras, which have less support.

STOPWATCH
Any mobile phone will have a stopwatch, and many apps will give you a vocalized countdown to zero.

HOW TO
WARM UP

*Even though the workouts are short, I always suggest that you warm up.
It will help make the workout more effective because you will be more flexible,
and you will then achieve a full range of motion through each move, which helps
get better results. Also, warming up helps to prevent any injuries.*

WARMING UP

To warm up, simply march on the spot for about 30 seconds (or longer if the weather is cold). If focusing on seated exercises, just do the arm moves if that suits you better. Once your body feels warm, you will be ready to work out. This helps prevent any injuries, while the increase in your core body temperature means your muscles become more pliable and flexible, so you get a much more efficient and effective workout.

HOW TO DO A DYNAMIC MARCH

Simply start marching on the spot, beginning with a light march, then progressing to march a little faster. Instead of swinging your arms back and forth, do big circles in front; this way you are mobilizing your upper and lower body. Aim to do this for 30 seconds, or, in the colder months, you may find you need to do it for up to 60 seconds to feel fully warmed up.

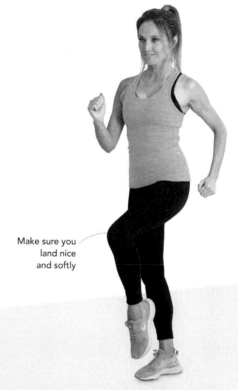

Make sure you land nice and softly

1 Start marching on the spot, gently at first, then progressing to lifting your knees up high and pumping your arms.

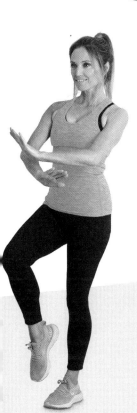

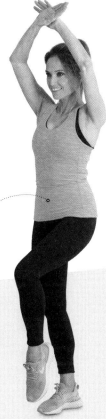

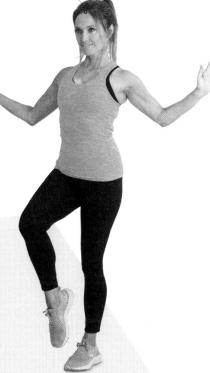

Tip

If you suffer tight muscles after working out, have a good long soak in the bath, then take a little longer warming up the next day.

Imagine big circles in your mind; this will help you create them ....

Keep your .... stomach muscles pulled in throughout, to aid stability

2 Still marching, mobilize your upper body by making circles in front of you with your arms.

3 Really reach your arms to their fullest as they circle in front of you, making the biggest circles you can.

4 Don't forget to carry on marching, while circling your arms. You'll feel your body warm up all over.

HOW TO

COOL DOWN & STRETCH

Once you have completed your 7-minute workout, you need to cool down. We are using very dynamic exercises with lateral moves that engage muscles you won't be used to working, so it's really important to stretch. To start with, simply march on the spot, or just use your marching arms, slowly bringing your heart rate and breathing back down to where they are when you are at rest. Then, perform these stretches. (Or, if you have been focusing on seated exercises, do the arm stretches on p24–25.)

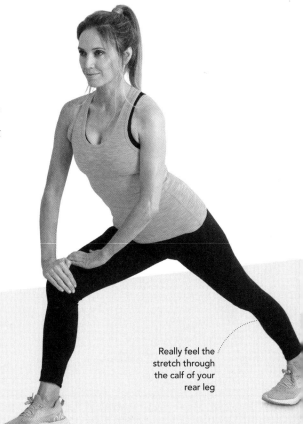

Tip

It's really important to do the stretches here and on p24–25 after working out. If you suffer aching muscles anyway, try going for a walk as well, to loosen up, and remember your muscles will get used to it.

Really feel the stretch through the calf of your rear leg

CALF STRETCH

Step back with one leg, keeping the heel down, both feet pointing forwards. Rest your hands on the bent leg. Lean into the stretch so you feel it in your calf. Hold for 10 seconds, then change to the other leg.

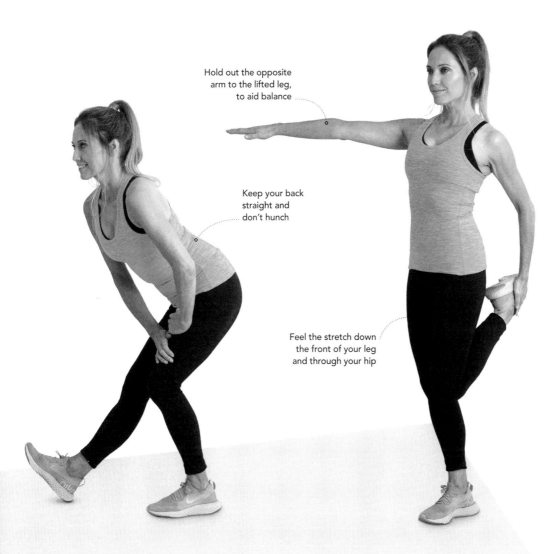

Hold out the opposite arm to the lifted leg, to aid balance

Keep your back straight and don't hunch

Feel the stretch down the front of your leg and through your hip

HAMSTRING STRETCH

Bend one leg and extend the other out straight in front of you, with your heel on the floor and your toes pointing up. Place both hands on the bent leg, and stick your bottom out to feel a stretch along the back of the straight leg. Hold for 20 seconds, then change to the other leg.

QUAD STRETCH

Standing with good posture, bend a leg behind you and gently hold the foot of the bent leg. Push your hips forward to feel the stretch in the front of your thigh. Keep the supporting knee slightly bent, or "soft". Hold for 10 seconds, then change to the other leg.

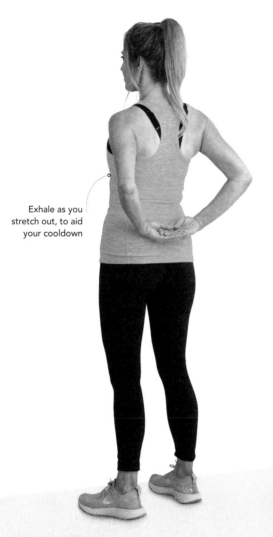

Exhale as you stretch out, to aid your cooldown

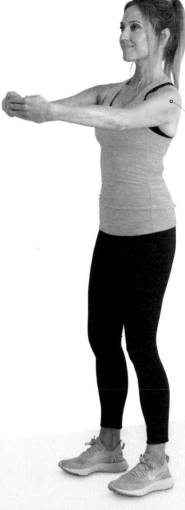

Keep your shoulders pulled down throughout the stretch

CHEST STRETCH

Stand with good posture, then take your arms behind you with your hands clasped together, and lift your shoulders up and back to feel the chest stretch. Hold for 10 seconds.

BACK STRETCH

Stand with good posture, knees soft, and tummy pulled in. Take your arms in front of you and imagine you are hugging a big beach ball. Feel the stretch in your back. Hold for 10 seconds.

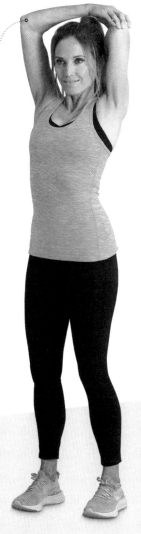

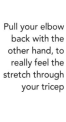

Pull your elbow back with the other hand, to really feel the stretch through your tricep

HEALTH & SAFETY

Before you do your 7-minute workout, it is always important to follow these rules for your safety.

The only times I advise you not to work out are:

- If you are feeling unwell
- If you have some form of injury
- If you have just eaten a big meal

But assuming you are good to go, then I would always recommend:

- Making sure you are hydrated and have some water with you.
- Always doing a quick warm-up (see p20–21).
- Making a point of listening to your body, and, if something does not feel right, stop.
- Doing the stretches I suggest (see this and the previous 2 pages) after your workout, to cool down.

TRICEP STRETCH
Lift 1 arm up and bend it behind your head, aiming to get your hand between your shoulder blades. Hold for 10 seconds. Then change to the other arm.

... And don't forget to go and record that you have completed another one of your workouts (see p30).

THE WORKOUTS

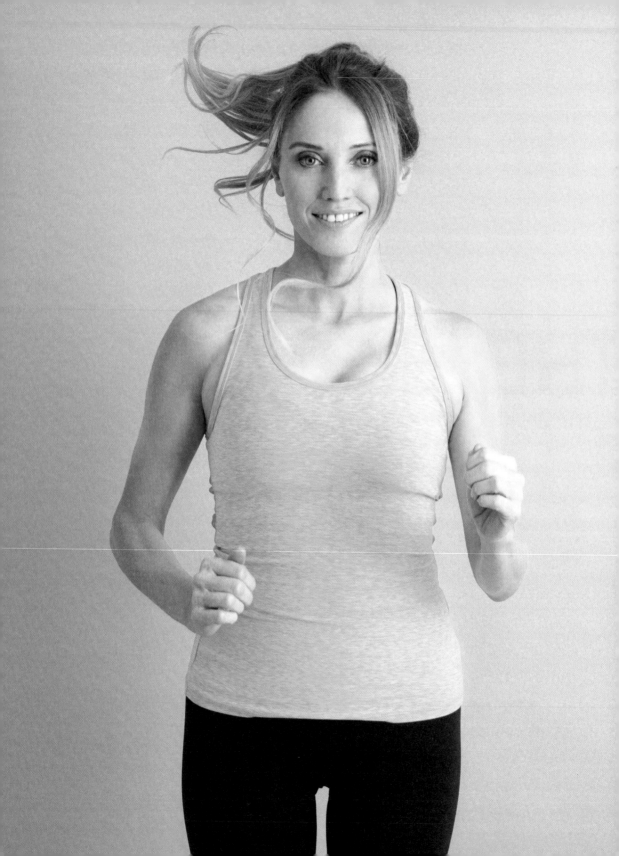

THE WORKOUTS

So here they are, my 7 workouts to do at home that will change the way you feel and get you maximum results: great health (the most important thing), a newly toned and sculpted body, and a positive mindset to keep you going on your fitness journey forever.

These workouts really are for everybody. You don't need to be a fitness fanatic, they are for people who want to improve their health and fitness levels wherever they are starting from. Use a wheelchair? Have a look at my Cardio-Boost & Sculpt Seated Workout (see p86). Just had a baby? You can work those abs, just go to p49 to see how to do it safely. Feeling unfit or overweight? Welcome! Your path to a fit body and a healthy weight starts here.

Each of the 7 workouts consists of 7 exercises, and each of those is just 60 seconds long. Try it for a week, really, commit to just that single week, and you'll be so amazed at the results that you'll carry on. To help track your progress, take a photo of the chart on p30 and fill it in every day. That will – I promise – encourage you to stick with it, if you're also following my 7 tips that maximize every workout's results (you'll find those at the end of each workout).

Most of the exercises – except for those in the seated workout, and a single move in the Melt off belly fat workout – are performed standing up. That is because, this way, you burn more calories, engage your muscles, and it makes it even easier to do it anytime, anywhere. In fact, I know from my social media feed how many people work out during their lunch hours!

I've also given you some FAQs, relevant to each workout, that I hope you will find useful, and will give you solutions to any questions you might have.

All my workouts will be effective however big (or small) the space you have available, or even if you are travelling. I've devised each and every exercise specifically to be performed in a small space and, despite that, all will give you brilliant results. You just need this book and, for one of the workouts, a cushion or a pillow. That's it.

So let's go. Turn the page for the most do-able and quickest way to a healthy body and mind.

7-DAY

CHECK LIST

Take a photo of this and print it out, then fill it in each week with your results. These could be measurements or timings; I'll tell you how to measure at the beginning of each workout.

WEEK 1 *Workout:* ....

DAY 1	DAY 2	DAY 3	DAY 4	DAY 5	DAY 6	DAY 7		before
								after

WEEK 2 *Workout:* ....

DAY 1	DAY 2	DAY 3	DAY 4	DAY 5	DAY 6	DAY 7		before
								after

WEEK 3 *Workout:* ....

DAY 1	DAY 2	DAY 3	DAY 4	DAY 5	DAY 6	DAY 7		before
								after

WEEK 4 *Workout:* ....

DAY 1	DAY 2	DAY 3	DAY 4	DAY 5	DAY 6	DAY 7		before
								after

WEEK 5 *Workout:* ....

DAY 1	DAY 2	DAY 3	DAY 4	DAY 5	DAY 6	DAY 7		before
								after

WEEK 6 *Workout:* ....

DAY 1	DAY 2	DAY 3	DAY 4	DAY 5	DAY 6	DAY 7		before
								after

WEEK 7 *Workout:* ....

DAY 1	DAY 2	DAY 3	DAY 4	DAY 5	DAY 6	DAY 7		before
								after

"Keep your
EYES FOCUSED ON
YOUR OWN JOURNEY
not the journeys
of others"

7-MINUTE

MELT OFF BELLY FAT WORKOUT

*This specially designed combination of 7 cardio-toning moves does 2 things: first, it reduces excess body fat by increasing calorie burn; second, it tones, tightens, and sculpts your waist. Many people think that, to work their abs, they have to do the plank, or sit-ups. But, to create curves, reduce tummy fat, and sculpt your waist, you get better results from standing up. Here, we work in all 3 directions the body is able to move in, especially rotationally, as this is what really hones the internal and external obliques (the muscles that draw in your waist). These are the 7 exercises that I used in the video that went viral (see p9) – and got thousands of amazing results for viewers. **They work!***

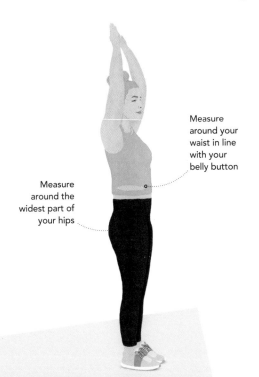

Measure around your waist in line with your belly button

Measure around the widest part of your hips

MEASURE YOUR PROGRESS

To track your results, grab a tape measure and wrap it around your waist in line with your belly button, just so you know in 7 days' time that you are measuring at the same point. I also suggest you measure around the widest part of your hips.

Tip

Take a picture on your phone of the 7-day checklist (see p30), then print it off, to record your progress.

OVERVIEW OF THE WORKOUT

Perform each move, flat out if you can, in the order shown for 1 minute. Don't forget to warm up and cool down (see p20–25).

MINUTE 1 — *The windmill*

MINUTE 2 — *The pendulum swing*

MINUTE 3 — *The walk down*

MINUTE 4 — *Speed skater lunge*

MINUTE 5 — *Sprinters' ab crunch*

MINUTE 6 — *Standing waist bends*

MINUTE 7 — *The ab makeover*

MINUTE 1

The windmill

In this full-body move, you engage your abs every time you kick your leg and bring your opposite arm forwards. Your tummy muscles jump into action, working to stabilize the core so you can keep your balance and alignment. Plus, you get the bonus of sculpting your arms and legs at the same time as increasing your metabolism, burning calories, and reducing body fat with each kick you take. And it is amazing at developing great hamstring flexibility. By day 7, you will find you can kick so much higher than you could on day 1.

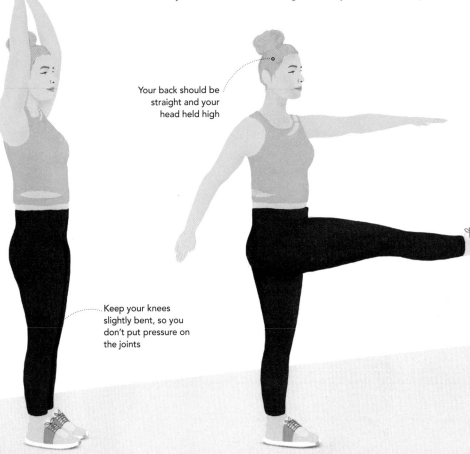

Your back should be straight and your head held high

Keep your knees slightly bent, so you don't put pressure on the joints

1 Stand straight with good posture, your feet hip-width apart, your chest lifted, and your shoulders pulled back. Lift your arms above your head and pull in your abs and glutes.

2 Kick one leg straight out in front of you, to a range of motion that is suitable for you, and at the same time bring your opposite arm towards the kicking foot.

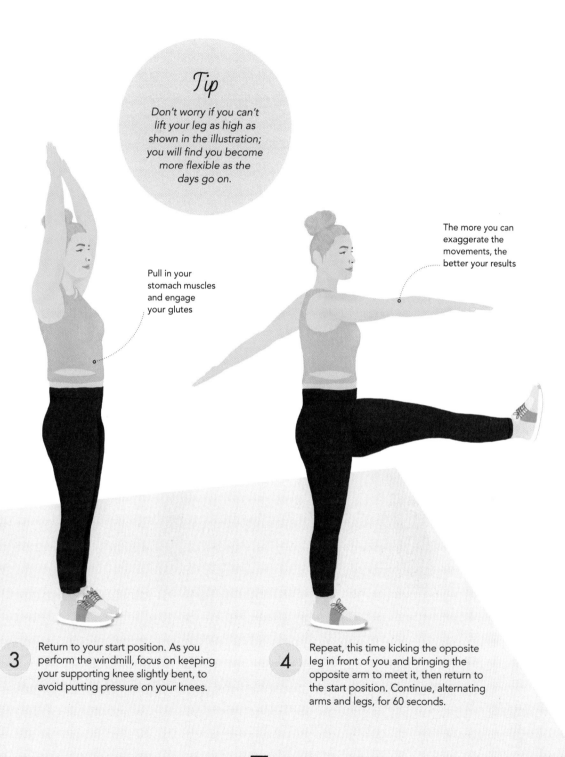

Tip

Don't worry if you can't lift your leg as high as shown in the illustration; you will find you become more flexible as the days go on.

Pull in your stomach muscles and engage your glutes

The more you can exaggerate the movements, the better your results

3 Return to your start position. As you perform the windmill, focus on keeping your supporting knee slightly bent, to avoid putting pressure on your knees.

4 Repeat, this time kicking the opposite leg in front of you and bringing the opposite arm to meet it, then return to the start position. Continue, alternating arms and legs, for 60 seconds.

MINUTE 2

The pendulum swing

This lateral move gets your heart rate up, working to strip off excess body fat, and it also activates your waist muscles as you transfer your body weight from one leg to the other. At the same time, you are working laterally (sideways), a range of motion that is often neglected, toning your inner and outer thighs, and you can actually feel your sides begin to tighten up as you swing. This full-body move may look amusing, but it will deliver some great results.

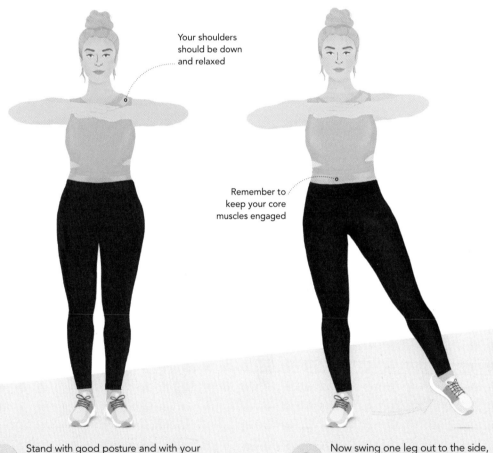

Your shoulders should be down and relaxed

Remember to keep your core muscles engaged

1 Stand with good posture and with your feet hip-width apart. Have your elbows bent and aiming to be at chest height, with your hands overlapping each other in front of you.

2 Now swing one leg out to the side, keeping your arms in the same position. Focus on keeping your hips facing forwards throughout.

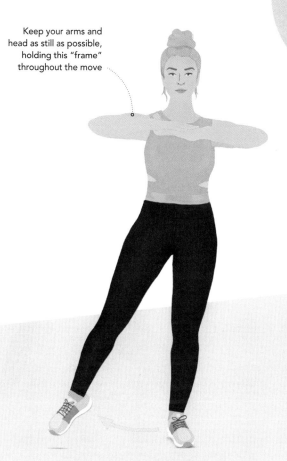

Keep your arms and head as still as possible, holding this "frame" throughout the move

Tip

If you would prefer a low-impact move, you can take out the jump and simply step it from side to side.

3 Bring the foot back and, at the same time, jump the other leg out to the other side. Alternate from side to side, for 60 seconds. Aim to land softly, to protect your joints.

MINUTE 3

The walk down

This travelling move may look easy, but it is a tough one. It engages all your major muscle groups: your arms, chest, and lower body. The exercise helps to activate calorie-burning muscle tissue throughout your body, so you continue to burn off more calories even after you've finished the workout. And guess what? Again, you should be fully engaging your abdominal muscles during this active exercise, especially if you are post-natal and have ab separation (*diastatis recti*). Perform this move slowly. Most people manage just 4–6 repetitions in 60 seconds.

Tip

If you find it too hard to come all the way down to the floor, do the move close to a sofa instead. Just lower your hands to your knees, then "walk" your hands out over the sofa, then "walk" them back in.

Engage your core muscles, especially if you have *diastatis recti*, while you walk down.

Once your hands are on the floor, don't bend your knees

1 Stand with good posture, with your arms raised directly above your head and your core muscles engaged.

2 Slowly start to "walk" your hands down your legs, bending your knees the lower you go, until your hands are on the ground. Now "walk" them out, until you come into a full push-up position.

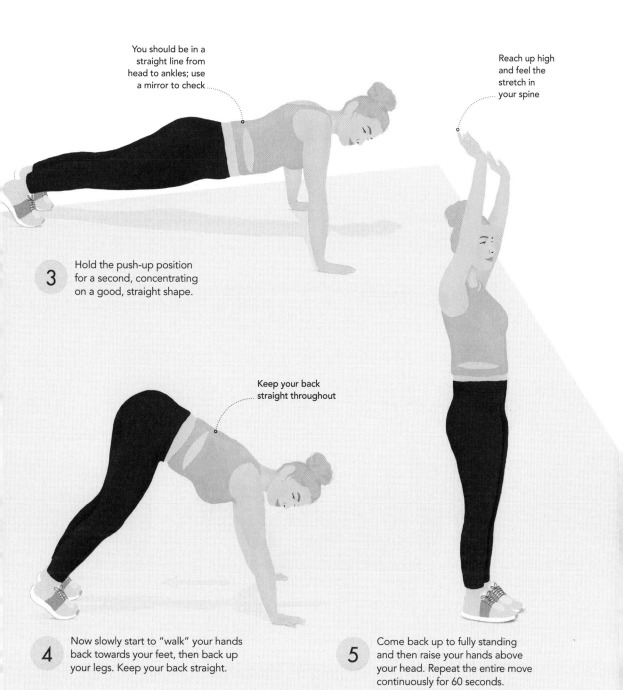

You should be in a straight line from head to ankles; use a mirror to check

Reach up high and feel the stretch in your spine

3 Hold the push-up position for a second, concentrating on a good, straight shape.

Keep your back straight throughout

4 Now slowly start to "walk" your hands back towards your feet, then back up your legs. Keep your back straight.

5 Come back up to fully standing and then raise your hands above your head. Repeat the entire move continuously for 60 seconds.

MINUTE 4

Speed skater lunge

This super-dynamic exercise is one of my personal favourite moves. You can just instantly feel the good it is doing you, and it is a superb way to create serious curves in your waist. Again, it's a total body calorie-burning move with bonus ab toning thrown in. Really exaggerate the lateral (sideways) movements here, bringing your arm all the way across your body until you can feel the stretch in your waist; that means your oblique muscles are kicking into action.

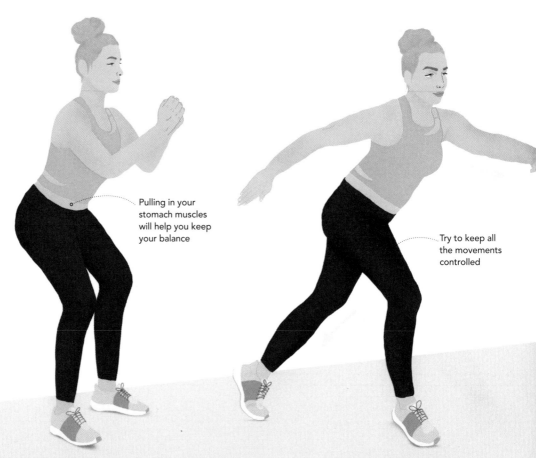

Pulling in your stomach muscles will help you keep your balance

Try to keep all the movements controlled

1 Start in a slight squat position, with your arms bent and in front of you. Remember: the bigger and deeper the move, the more calories you burn, and the more toned you become.

2 Now jump one foot behind and across your front leg and at the same time bring the same side arm across as far as you can, keeping it at chest height, with the other arm out behind you.

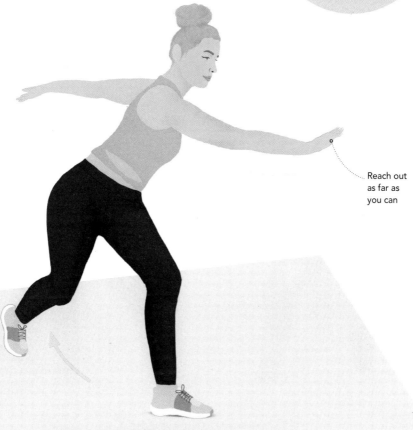

Tip

If you find the jumping hard, you can turn this into a low-impact exercise by simply stepping from side to side rather than jumping.

Reach out as far as you can

3 Then switch to the leg and arm on the other side, as if you're ice skating. Alternate from side to side. Each time, aim to get the hand as far over to the side as you can, and the leg deep behind, for maximum results. Repeat, alternating sides, for 60 seconds.

MINUTE 5

Sprinters' ab crunch

This exercise really shows that the best way to get fab results is to do standing ab moves. You will feel it working instantly, literally sprinting off excess body fat and defining, sculpting, and strengthening your abs. Also, it is amazing at sculpting your glutes and toning your arms: bonus. Note that, for this exercise, you spend 30 seconds on one leg, then change to the other leg for the final 30 seconds.

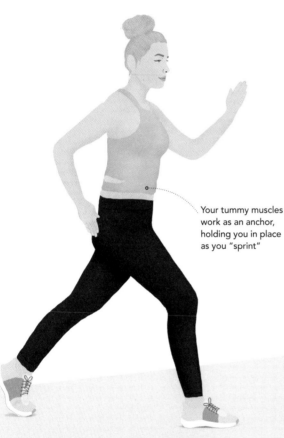

Your tummy muscles work as an anchor, holding you in place as you "sprint"

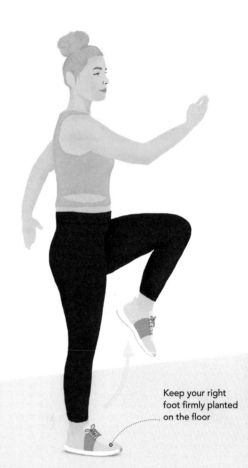

Keep your right foot firmly planted on the floor

1 Start in a split position: bend both arms at the elbows, slightly bend your knees, then bring your left leg behind you and your left arm in front of you. Your weight should be on your right leg, and your right arm behind you.

2 Now imagine you are about to sprint: drive your left knee (the one behind you) forwards and up and your left arm directly behind, while your right arm comes forward.

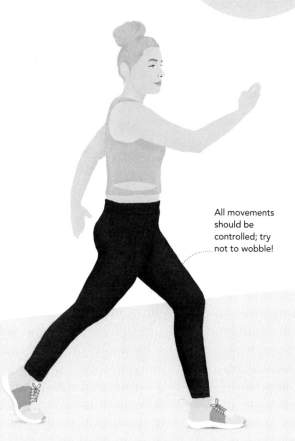

All movements should be controlled; try not to wobble!

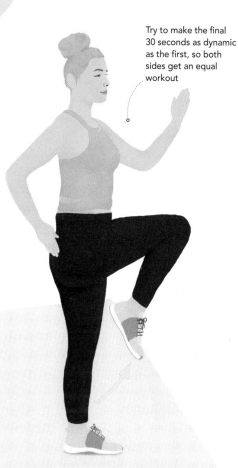

Try to make the final 30 seconds as dynamic as the first, so both sides get an equal workout

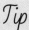

3 Now step it back, keeping your weight on the right foot. Staying on the same side, keep repeating the move for 30 seconds. Focus on keeping your tummy muscles pulled in as tight as you can throughout.

4 After 30 seconds, change sides and transfer your weight to your left foot. Keep repeating crunches on this side for the final 30 seconds of the move, even though you will be getting tired.

MINUTE 6

Standing waist bends

A lovely, graceful, low-impact move that focuses a little more on the arms and abs. Again, we are still working through a big range of motion, so this helps to keep that calorie burn nice and high at the same time as shaping through your waist. Notice that we are again working laterally (sideways) here, to achieve the results we want in the waist area. This exercise will also improve your flexibility.

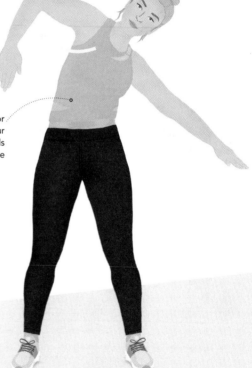

Perform the move as if someone was watching, to keep it graceful and smooth

Don't twist or lean over; keep your body facing forwards throughout the move

1 Stand with your feet slightly wider than shoulder-width apart, your feet pointing out at a 45-degree angle, and your knees slightly bent. Have your arms crossed over your chest.

2 Keeping your lower body still, uncross your arms, and reach one arm out as far as you can to one side, extending that arm straight and down. The other arm should stay bent and lift up higher. Hold for a second and you should feel the stretch through your waist.

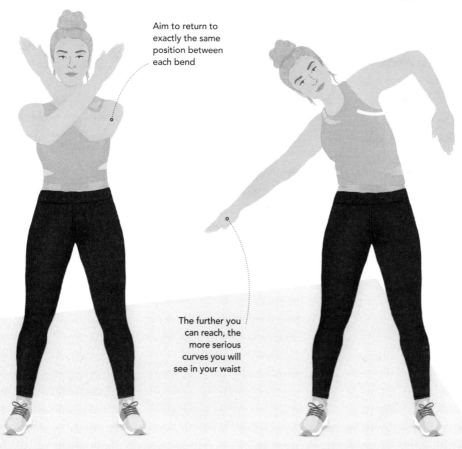

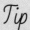

Tip

Always move as far as you can, to ensure you get maximum results.

Aim to return to exactly the same position between each bend

The further you can reach, the more serious curves you will see in your waist

3 Now come back to your starting position, crossing your arms again, still keeping your lower body still and your knees slightly bent.

4 Now uncross your arms, reaching out to the opposite side; again reach out as far as you can so you feel it in your waist. Focus on keeping your hips still throughout the move. Alternate the waist bends for 60 seconds.

MINUTE 7

The ab makeover

We come down on to the floor for a nice way to end this 7-minute workout. This ab move is super-powerful and targets your entire mid-section, as well as working a little bit through your legs. Though you are on the floor, this exercise will still keep your heart rate up.

Tip

If it's too hard to do this move on the floor, or if you are post-natal and have diastasis recti (ab separation), it is better to skip this move. Simply repeat Minute 1 "The Windmill" until you have healed.

Try not to strain your neck; you should remain comfortable throughout the exercise

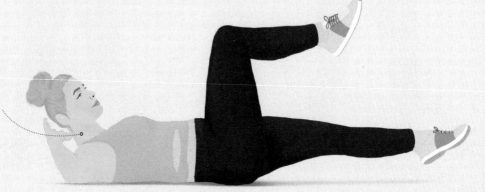

1 Lie on the floor, face up, hands by the side of your head, and lift your head from the floor. Have one leg fully extended and several inches off the ground, and the other bent.

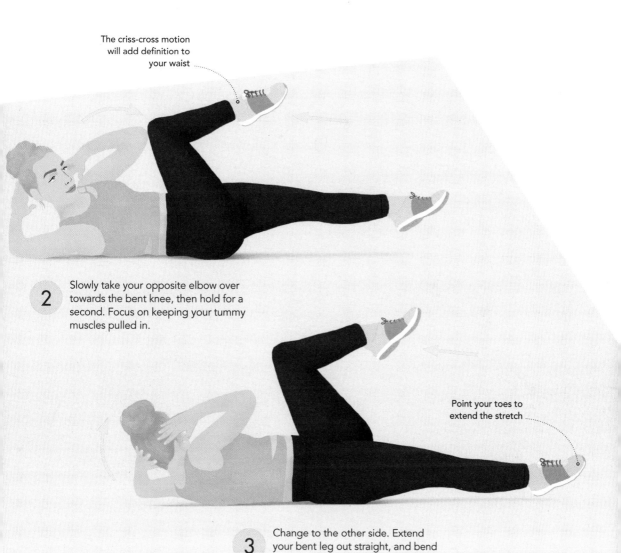

The criss-cross motion will add definition to your waist

2 Slowly take your opposite elbow over towards the bent knee, then hold for a second. Focus on keeping your tummy muscles pulled in.

Point your toes to extend the stretch

3 Change to the other side. Extend your bent leg out straight, and bend the straight leg in. Bring the opposite elbow across towards the bent knee. Keep alternating from side to side for 60 seconds.

TO HELP GET THAT FLAT BELLY

7 TIPS

1 BAN THE BLOAT.

Obviously, food plays a big part in the appearance of our tummies! As with all the 7-minute challenges, I stress that to get the best results you must focus on good nutrition and correct portion sizes (see p138). But some healthy choices can cause bloating, giving us a "food baby". If you find this happens to you, here are some of the likely suspects... and some good alternatives to try instead.

BLOATERS	REPLACE WITH
beans	grains, meat, fish
lentils	quinoa, couscous
carbonated drinks	water, herbal teas
wheat cereals	pure oats
broccoli, cauliflower, cabbage, sprouts	spinach, cucumber, sweet potato, lettuce
raw onion	herbs and spices
dairy milk, cheese, yogurt	dairy-free options, such as almond, soya (soy), or rice milk
apples	bananas, oranges, strawberries

FAQ

What is the best way to get rid of belly fat?

A combination of being consistent with fat-burning exercise, and performing sculpting moves for your waist, alongside healthy eating. For best results, you need a large range of motion. This is why, in my Melt off belly fat workout, I have you standing up, because then – instead of just using a couple of muscles – you are recruiting hundreds to help. As a result, you are burning serious amounts of calories. Standing exercises are always going to be your best bet.

2 BE SUGAR-SMART.

If you buy pre-packaged food, *read the label*. The further up the list sugar appears, the more a product contains.

In the UK, a low-sugar product is defined as containing 5g (⅙oz) total sugars per 100g (3½oz). A high-sugar product contains 22.5g (¾oz) total sugars per 100g (3½oz).

Don't assume that because an item is savoury it won't contain sugar; it's even added to prawns and shrimp! So, for optimal health, eat food that is not pre-packaged. If you do buy prepared foods, aim for low-sugar products.

3 GET UP!

When we sit for long periods, our clever bodies realize we require less energy. So they reduce the amount of calories we burn. A good analogy is to imagine you are sitting in a car in a traffic jam not going anywhere. You would turn the engine off. Well, this is what our metabolic system does. So, to keep that engine running, get up every 20 minutes and walk around, even just to get a glass of water, to keep your calorie burn higher.

4 TONE IT UP ON YOUR COMMUTE.

Try the secret exercise below. I am all about time-saving ways to get results. You can do this on your commute, sitting or standing: nobody will know.

The Discreet Tummy Toner. Picture your belly button. Now imagine you have to pull it in as tight as you can towards your spine. Hold for several seconds, then release and repeat.

This strengthens and defines your *transverse abdominis*, a corset-shaped muscle. The more you do it, the more you sculpt your waist, and the stronger the core muscles become.

5 GET TO BED BEFORE 10:30PM.

Having 7 hours of good-quality sleep helps control your hormones. If you get fewer than 7 hours, you can confuse feeling tired with being hungry, which is why we crave carb-rich food after a bad night's sleep (or a night partying).

6 DRINK UP.

Water is a must when you want to achieve your best abs. By keeping fully hydrated, your metabolism stays working flat-out. Water keeps you feeling full, it keeps you energized, and it reduces constipation and bloating. Have a large glass before every meal.

7 MINDFUL EATING.

If you eat on the go – breakfast in the car, lunch at your desk, or dinner doing emails – it can often mean you don't appreciate what you're eating. Take time out to sit down and eat without distractions, and eat slowly, instead of "inhaling" food on the go.

FAQ

I had a baby 3 months ago. Is this workout safe to do, as I still have a gap from diastasis recti.

You can adapt this workout to be *diastasis recti*-friendly. Keep your core muscles engaged throughout move 3 "The Walk Down" (see p38). Also replace move 7 with move 1 "The Windmill" (see p34). This makes it a safe workout for you and will even help to repair your abdominal separation more rapidly.

7-MINUTE

DREAM ARMS WORKOUT

Get ready to shrug off your cardigan and feel T-shirt confident with this 7-minute workout. Whether you call them "bingo wings", "aunty arms", or "lunch-lady arms", this is often a troublesome area for women, where we tend to store fat and lose muscle tone. But, with the right exercises, we can address any problems and start shaping and sculpting to give you the confidence to go sleeveless.
For this workout I am focusing on 2 aspects: the first is cardio, to get your heart rate up, helping to reduce your overall body fat; the second is arm sculpting, toning through your arms, shoulders, and overall upper body. And, at the same time, we will be improving your upper body strength and your posture.

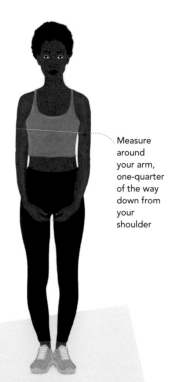

Measure around your arm, one-quarter of the way down from your shoulder

MEASURE YOUR PROGRESS

There are a couple of tests you can do. You can do both or just one, the choice is yours.

METHOD 1 – INCH LOSS RESULTS
Grab a tape measure and measure around your left arm (or right arm, if you are left-handed), one-quarter of the way down from your shoulder. Repeat on the last day of the workout.

METHOD 2 – ENDURANCE RESULTS
Warm up (see p20), then do a press-up (push-up). If you are a beginner, start with your knees on the ground (the "boxed version"). If you're more experienced, try a full press-up. Do this on days 1 and 7 to see your strength improve.

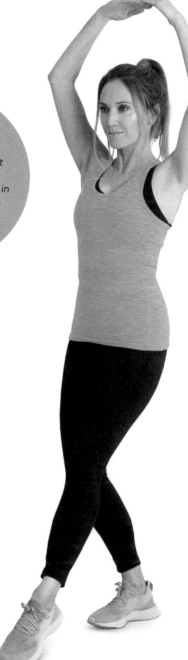

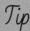

Tip

This workout is all about reaching, so, in every exercise, try to keep that in mind, and really stretch those arms as far as they will go.

OVERVIEW OF THE WORKOUT

Perform each move, flat out if you can, in the order shown for 1 minute. Don't forget to warm up and cool down (see p20–25).

MINUTE 1 *Marching arms*

MINUTE 2 *Arm definer*

MINUTE 3 *Go sleeveless punch*

MINUTE 4 *Skip to sculpt*

MINUTE 5 *T-shirt tone arms*

MINUTE 6 *Ballerina arms*

MINUTE 7 *Tricep reach to the sky*

MINUTE 1

Marching arms

As well as working to sculpt your arms, this move is amazing at helping you to naturally give your bust a boost. This is because it tightens Cooper's ligament, which I call "Nature's bra strap". (To read more about it, see p66.)

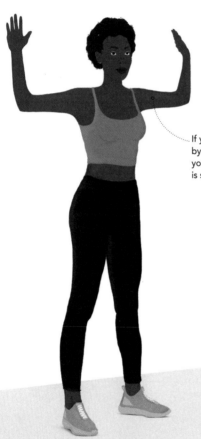

If you can exercise by a mirror, check your movement is symmetrical

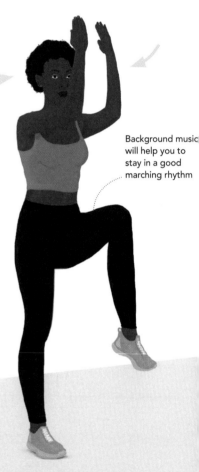

Background music will help you to stay in a good marching rhythm

1 Standing with good upright posture and with your feet hip-width apart, bend your arms and bring them out to your sides, your elbows in line with your shoulders and each forming a right angle, with your palms facing forwards.

2 Start marching on the spot, then bring both your arms in to the centre, so your palms touch and your forearms are in parallel. Keep your belly button pulled in towards your spine.

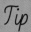

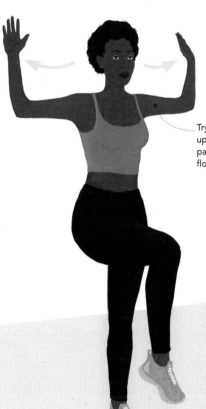

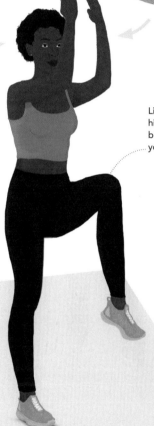

Try to keep your upper arms parallel to the floor at all times

Lift your knee as high as you can, but don't lose your balance

3 Open your arms back out, while still marching on the spot. Be careful to touch your foot softly on the ground, to protect your joints.

4 Continue the move for 60 seconds. As usual, the more you move, the greater the benefits, so lift your kneesß as high as you can and keep your elbows in line with your shoulders throughout.

MINUTE 2

Arm definer

This move is amazing at really targeting the back of the upper arms – that area often referred to as "aunty arms" (poor aunty!) – while adding the leg kick helps us to reduce excess fat by adding cardio to the sculpting here. At the same time, the kick includes more muscles in the move, thus increasing your overall calorie burn.

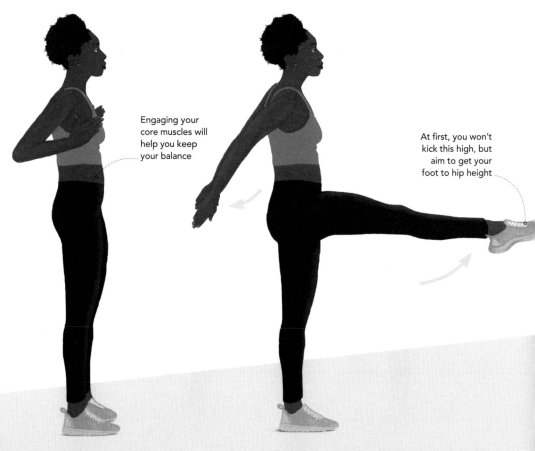

Engaging your core muscles will help you keep your balance

At first, you won't kick this high, but aim to get your foot to hip height

1 Stand with good posture, arms bent, and elbows lifted and behind you. Your thumbs should be by your shoulders and your palms facing in.

2 Now kick one leg out in front of you and, at the same time, straighten your arms back, reaching behind as far as you can.

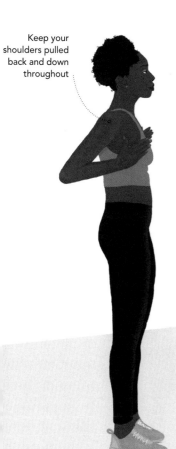

Keep your shoulders pulled back and down throughout

Reach far enough back that you really feel the stretch in your arms and shoulders

Tip

Focus on keeping your elbows lifted as high as you can behind you, while still being comfortable.

3 Bring your leg and arms back to the starting position. Remember to keep pulling your tummy muscles in and to land softly on your feet.

4 Now kick the opposite leg in front and repeat the same arm movement. Keep alternating leg kicks for 60 seconds.

MINUTE 3

Go sleeveless punch

This move will not only give you amazing toned arms, but it is fantastic for sculpting and toning your waist at the same time. Try to reach as far out to each side as you possibly can with every punch, to gain the maximum results.

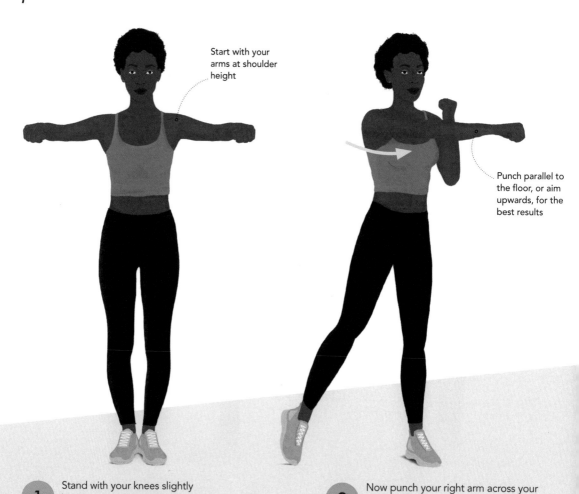

Start with your arms at shoulder height

Punch parallel to the floor, or aim upwards, for the best results

1 Stand with your knees slightly bent, your arms bent to the sides, and your fists pointing forwards.

2 Now punch your right arm across your body as far as you can go, stepping your right foot out to the side at the same time, so you can get a really deep punch.

Exhaling sharply as you punch can make the movement more powerful

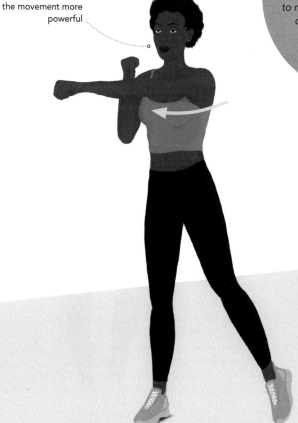

Tip

As you transfer your weight from one leg to the other, you can add in a slight jump, to make it a little harder. Also, to challenge your arms more, punch higher up. This instantly makes your arms work harder.

3 Now punch the left arm across and step out the left leg. Keep punching from side to side for 60 seconds, and remember to reach as far as you can.

MINUTE 4

Skip to sculpt

This is great for your arms, but also amazing for strengthening and sculpting through your shoulders. It's a cardio move that gets your heart pumping and burns calories for hours after the workout is over. Skipping is an excellent way to tone up and lose fat, while giving you those enviable arms. You don't even need a rope for this move!

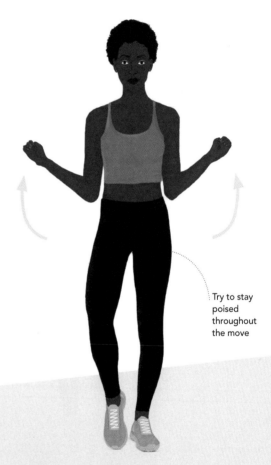

Tip

The bigger you make the arm movements, the more challenging this exercise becomes. If you happen to have a skipping rope handy, you could always do this for real.

Try to stay poised throughout the move

1. Stand with good posture and imagine you are holding a skipping rope (jump rope), so have your arms slightly bent and raised to your sides.

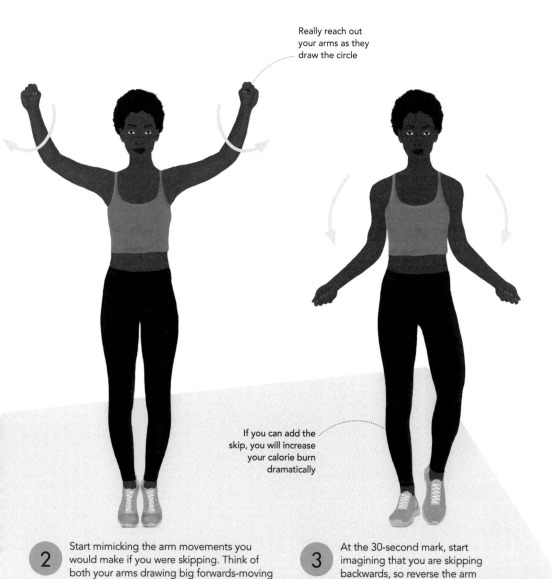

Really reach out your arms as they draw the circle

If you can add the skip, you will increase your calorie burn dramatically

2 Start mimicking the arm movements you would make if you were skipping. Think of both your arms drawing big forwards-moving circles. At the same time, march on the spot, or – if you want to work a little harder – you can take it from a light march to a skip.

3 At the 30-second mark, start imagining that you are skipping backwards, so reverse the arm rotation for the final 30 seconds.

MINUTE 5

T-shirt tone arms

This helps to sculpt that area at the back of the upper arms which can often be the first to lose definition. Don't worry, because this move will bring it back. But don't be fooled, this exercise is far harder than it looks, so be prepared for a challenge. For the best results, try to keep your upper arms parallel to the floor throughout the move.

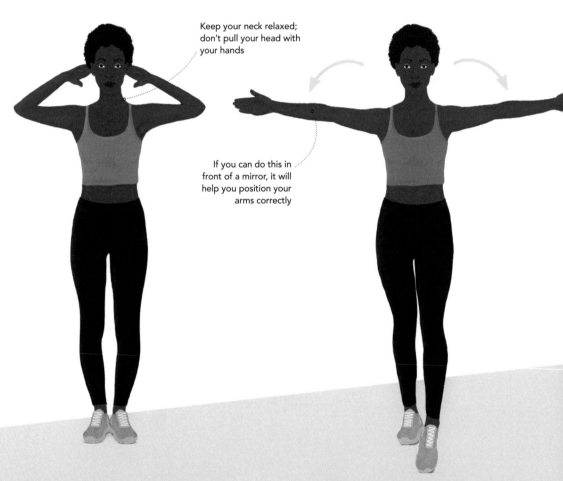

Keep your neck relaxed; don't pull your head with your hands

If you can do this in front of a mirror, it will help you position your arms correctly

1 Stand with good posture. Slightly bend your knees to prevent locking the joints. Place your fingertips by the side of your head and your arms out to the sides, keeping your elbows at shoulder height.

2 Now straighten your arms out and hold for a second, so your body looks like the letter "T", tapping your right foot out in front of you. Focus on keeping your upper arms parallel to the floor.

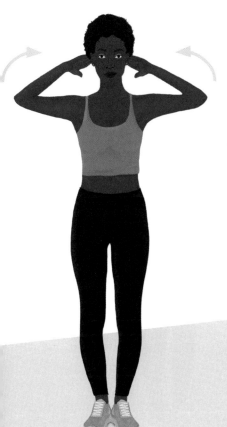

Tip

If you need to rest your arms for a few seconds, that is fine, but – as you progress through the 7 days – you'll find it gets easier. You can move your feet and do a slight march at the same time if you wish (it may distract from the arm burn).

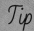

Try to work as hard during the last 5 seconds as you did at the start

March with high knees, for an added cardio bonus

3 Now bend your arms back to the start position, still remembering to keep those upper arms parallel to the floor. Bring your right foot back in at the same time.

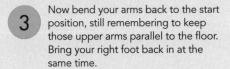

4 Open up your arms once more, to form that letter "T", tapping your left foot out in front of you. Carry on for 60 seconds. You can do it!

MINUTE 6
Ballerina arms

This move is as graceful as it sounds, and it fits perfectly into the sequence for this 7-minute routine, especially after the previous exercise. It will help to define your arms and shoulders beautifully and, at the same time, give your inner thighs a little workout, too.

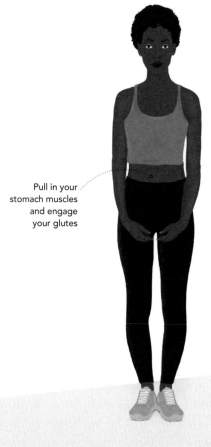

Pull in your stomach muscles and engage your glutes

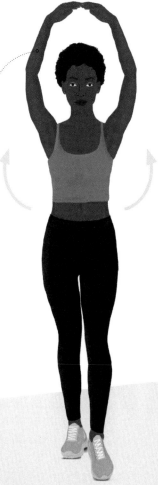

Try to keep a beautifully rounded shape in both arms

1 Stand with good posture, with your feet close together, your arms relaxed with a slight bend in the elbow and resting on the front of your thighs. Your hands should be cupped with the palms facing upwards.

2 Now point one foot in front, slightly turned out at a 45-degree angle. At the same time, keeping your fingertips close, lift both arms above your head, then hold.

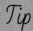

Tip

As you lift and lower your arms, imagine that they are resisting against a weight on the way up and the way down; this is where we can really use our minds to help increase the intensity of an exercise.

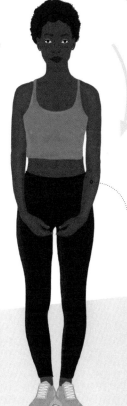

Keep all the movements slow, smooth, and deliberate

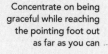

Concentrate on being graceful while reaching the pointing foot out as far as you can

3 Lower your arms back down to the start position and bring your foot back in. Focus on keeping your balance, and hold yourself with excellent posture.

4 Now lift your arms back up and point the opposite foot in front, again remembering to point it out at a 45-degree angle. Continue, alternating legs, for 60 seconds.

MINUTE 7

Tricep reach to the sky

This move is very specific to targeting the back of your upper arms, working hard on getting a lovely tone and sculpt through that common problem area. At the beginning of the 7 days, you might find that your hands will not touch your upper back, but as you progress through the week, you should find that your flexibility will improve.

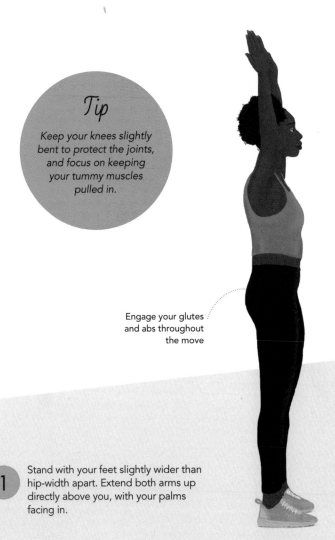

Tip

Keep your knees slightly bent to protect the joints, and focus on keeping your tummy muscles pulled in.

Engage your glutes and abs throughout the move

1 Stand with your feet slightly wider than hip-width apart. Extend both arms up directly above you, with your palms facing in.

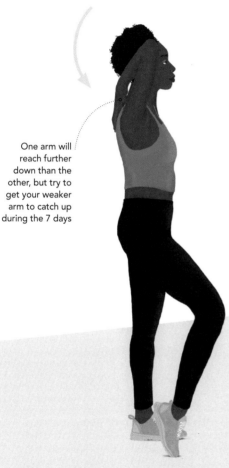

The higher you can reach your arms, the better your results

One arm will reach further down than the other, but try to get your weaker arm to catch up during the 7 days

2 Now bend your arms at the elbows, aiming for your fingertips to touch the top of your upper back. Reach down as far as you can.

3 Now extend the arms back up to your start position. Repeat for 60 seconds. If you like, you could also add a ballerina foot (see p62).

TO HELP GET THOSE DREAM ARMS

7 TIPS

1 CUP OF TEA WITH A PRESS-UP.
Every time you are waiting for the tea to brew, lean into the work surface with your feet about 15cm (6in) away and do a few press-ups (push-ups). Keep your legs straight, but don't lock your knees, to protect the joints. This exercise will help tone your arms and upper body. It will also help to tighten "Nature's bra strap" (see FAQ, below).

2 SPEED UP YOUR WALKS.
When we walk faster we naturally use our arms more, as the piston action helps propel us forwards faster. So on your way to work, or whenever you are out and about walking, add some intervals at a slightly faster pace, combined with those pumping arms, to give the arms a little bit of an extra sculpt while you walk. For the best results, exaggerate the action.

3 USE SHOPPING BASKETS.
OK, if you are on a big shopping trip, use a trolley, but, for a quicker trip, go for 2 baskets instead, one on each arm. Once you start filling those up with healthy fruits and vegetables, it will give your arms a great workout. Don't hold back: get as much as you can carry! And if your supermarket is reasonably close to home, carry the groceries home by yourself, too, rather than taking the car. (That's not always possible, but it's great if you can manage it.)

4 BAN THE JUNK.
If you really want to reduce arm fat, then to help you get the maximum results during this 7 days I have one simple tip: don't buy any junk food,

FAQ

My bust has started to sag, can I help give it a natural lift?

The culprit is Cooper's ligament, connective tissue that lifts the bust. It is attached to your collar bone and pectorals, so over time it becomes loose and stretched, which makes our breasts sag. If you tighten the ligament then – hey presto! – you can have a firm and lifted bust again. Great exercises for toning this area are a press-up (push-up), or a Marching arm sculptor (see p52).

sugary snacks, or processed foods. If you haven't got them in the kitchen cupboards, you can't eat them. And avoid the sugary snacks at work, too. Stock up with herbal tea, so you can sip on it, rehydrate, and fill up, avoiding the temptation to snack. Plus, look at my Healthy Snacks (see pp182–191), for when the between-meal urge gets too strong to resist.

5 SWIM WHILE THE ADS ARE ON.

This is a fun one, but a great way to tone your arms while watching TV. Simply mimic a swimming action during every ad break. As ever, exaggerate the movements of the arms as you perform a "breast stroke". If you're feeling energetic, you could even get down on your front, lift your arms and legs off the floor, and perform a full body "swim".

6 SHAKE IT OUT.

Every morning, when you get up and make your bed, lift up your duvet to give it a few good shakes. Do it again in the evening, before you hop between the sheets. The stronger and more vigorous the movements here, the better. This is a similar motion to one commonly used in gym weights rooms, shaking out "battle ropes". So make it a habit and do it as often as you remember.

FAQ

Can you really get fit at home, or do you need to go to a gym?

Yes, you can get in the best shape of your life at home, without any equipment. Your body is your own gym and you don't need weights; in my workouts, you use your own body weight. The great thing with home fitness is that it so easily becomes a lifestyle, so – no excuses – everyone can get fit at home, whether you are a beginner, intermediate, or any age or ability.

7 UPLIFTING ARM SCRUB.

When we feel good about ourselves, it is easier to stay on track, so as our goal this week is to get your arms looking and feeling good, give this home-made arm-moisturizing scrub a try.

What you need:
1 tsp sea salt flakes
1 tbsp coconut oil
several drops of peppermint oil

Mix everything together, then, in the shower or bath, gently rub on your arms, starting from your hands and working up to your shoulders, making sure the mix is fully absorbed. Rinse off. Your arms should feel silky-smooth.

7-MINUTE

LOVE MY LEGS WORKOUT

You use your legs from the moment you step out of bed, and they carry you around all day, but mostly through what's known as the Sagittal plane of motion (forward and back). The other two planes are Frontal (lateral moves), and Transverse (rotational). If you use just the Sagittal plane, you are missing out on toning and sculpting your inner and outer thigh muscles. Therefore, to get gorgeous legs and sculpt and tighten them, you need to target the muscles down their sides. So I have the perfect combination of 7 moves that are going to target all your leg muscles and from lots of angles, so you will see great results.

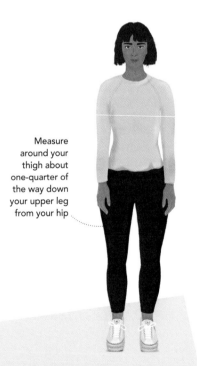

Measure around your thigh about one-quarter of the way down your upper leg from your hip

MEASURE YOUR PROGRESS

There are a couple of tests you can do. You can do both or just one, the choice is yours.

METHOD 1 – INCH LOSS RESULTS

To measure your results, find a tape measure and wrap it around your left thigh one-quarter of the way down your upper leg from your hip.

METHOD 2 – ENDURANCE RESULTS

Warm up (see p20). Perform alternating lunges (see p110), doing as many as you can. As soon as they start to feel challenging, note the number you were able to do. The day after you have completed the 7-day challenge, redo this test.

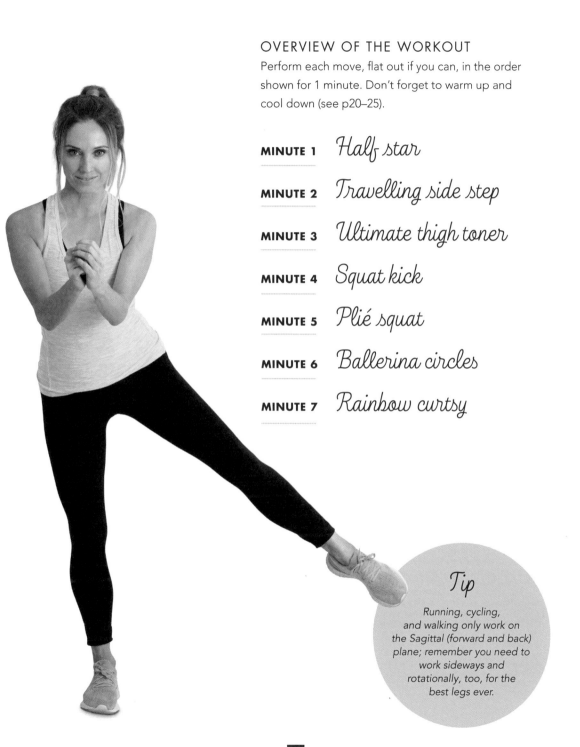

OVERVIEW OF THE WORKOUT

Perform each move, flat out if you can, in the order shown for 1 minute. Don't forget to warm up and cool down (see p20–25).

MINUTE 1 *Half star*

MINUTE 2 *Travelling side step*

MINUTE 3 *Ultimate thigh toner*

MINUTE 4 *Squat kick*

MINUTE 5 *Plié squat*

MINUTE 6 *Ballerina circles*

MINUTE 7 *Rainbow curtsy*

Tip

Running, cycling, and walking only work on the Sagittal (forward and back) plane; remember you need to work sideways and rotationally, too, for the best legs ever.

MINUTE 1
Half star

This exercise is great for getting your heart rate up, so you are actively burning a high amount of calories. At the same time, because it is a Frontal (lateral) move (see p68), you are targeting the outer thigh muscles. You may wonder why you are using arms in a leg workout; the simple reason is that by bringing in the arm movement, this leg exercise becomes a great fat-burning move, too.

Tip

Be sure to step each foot out as far to the side as possible, as this will keep the intensity of the exercise nice and high.

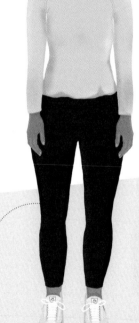

Don't lock your knee joints; keep them nice and soft

1 Stand straight with good posture, your arms relaxed, and your palms resting on the front of your thighs.

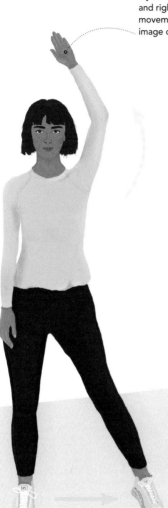

Try to keep your left- and right-hand movements the mirror image of each other

Feel the stretch down your active side with each repeated move

2 Now lift your left arm directly up and, at the same time, lift the left leg out to the side.

3 Now repeat on the right-hand side, lifting your right arm and leg. Keep alternating from side to side.

MINUTE 2

Travelling side step

This is great for building endurance in your lower body, as the extended squat works all the muscles in your legs. Plus, taking a big side step means you are working your body through the Frontal (lateral) plane of motion (see p68), which will help to tone and sculpt your thighs.

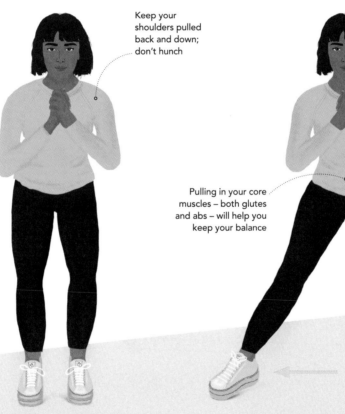

Keep your shoulders pulled back and down; don't hunch

Pulling in your core muscles – both glutes and abs – will help you keep your balance

1 Start by coming into a low squat position, knees bent, arms bent, and hands together. Get as low as you can.

2 Now, staying low, simply step your left foot out to the side, taking a big, deep side step.

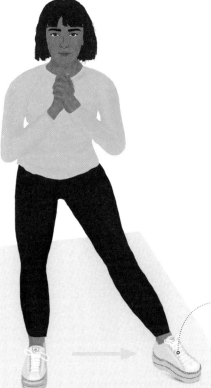

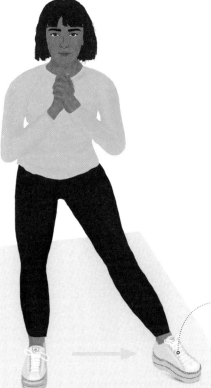

Tip

The lower you bend down into the move, the harder it becomes and the better your results.

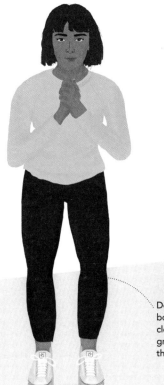

Don't let your body rise up; stay close to the ground during this move

Be sure to keep taking wide, deep steps

3 Still staying low, bring the right leg close to the left foot. Step the left foot out wide again. If you have enough space, travel 4 steps. If you are tighter on space, just do 2 steps.

4 Travel back the other way for another 2 or 4 steps. Focus on keeping your body as low as you can throughout, to maximize results..

MINUTE 3
Ultimate thigh toner

This move is working on both your standing leg and on the active leg. You get to engage lots of muscles in the standing leg that help to stabilize your body, which is naturally great for improving your balance. Plus, this exercise includes a leg lift, which is going to streamline your thighs, giving them some great definition.

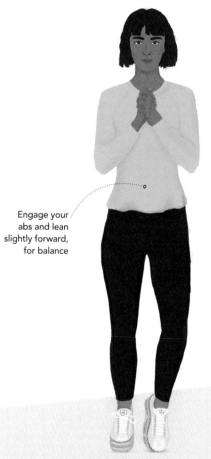

Engage your abs and lean slightly forward, for balance

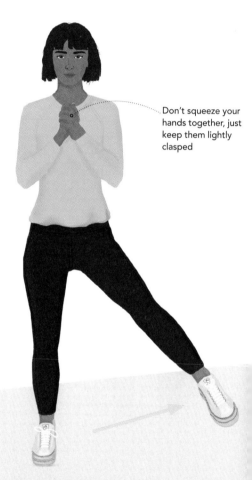

Don't squeeze your hands together, just keep them lightly clasped

1 Stand with a slight bend in both legs, with good posture, your arms bent and hands lightly clasped, and leaning slightly forward.

2 Keeping your weight on your right leg, lift your left leg out to the side, as high as feels comfortable. Hold for a second, then allow the foot to lightly touch the floor, before lifting it straight back up. Keep repeating this, tapping with the same leg for 30 seconds.

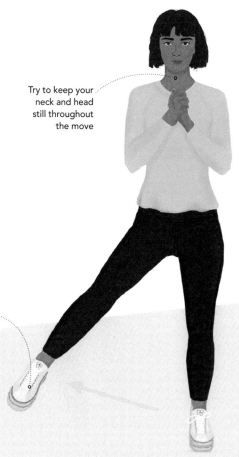

Try to keep your neck and head still throughout the move

Tip

Keep the range of movement controlled. Avoid swinging your leg so high that you turn your hips out.

Try to make your last leg lift as high as the first

3 Change to the other leg for the final 30 seconds. Lift it as high as possible each time, and just tap the floor with your foot softly.

MINUTE 4

Squat kick

This move is going to lift, tone, and sculpt your entire lower body. It will also help to get your heart rate up, as it is a massively calorie-burning move. Plus it is fabulous at toning your backside, too. It is quite a difficult exercise, with a big range of motion, but even if you find it hard at the beginning of the 7 days, I bet it will get easier for you over the week.

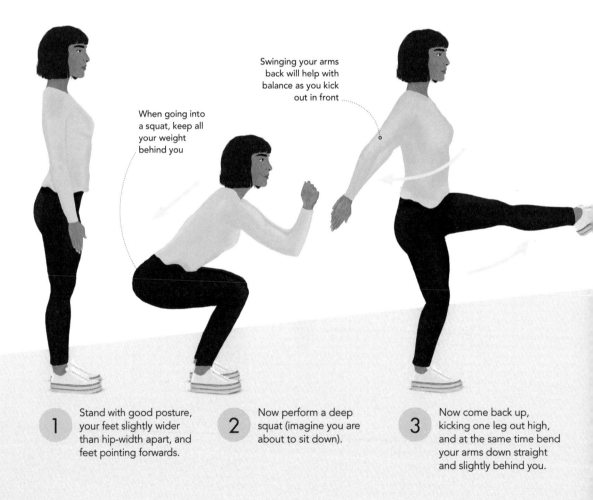

When going into a squat, keep all your weight behind you

Swinging your arms back will help with balance as you kick out in front

1   Stand with good posture, your feet slightly wider than hip-width apart, and feet pointing forwards.

2   Now perform a deep squat (imagine you are about to sit down).

3   Now come back up, kicking one leg out high, and at the same time bend your arms down straight and slightly behind you.

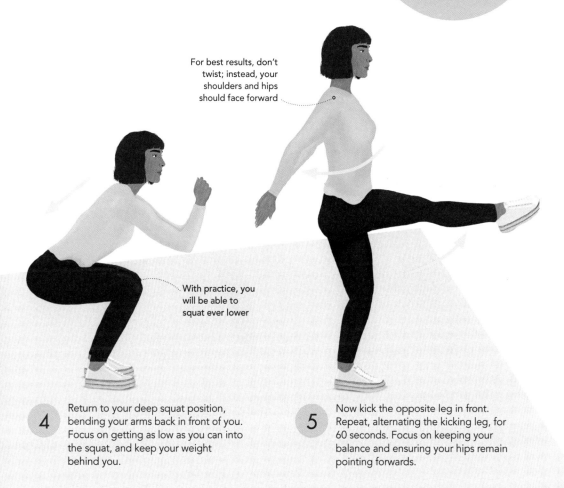

For best results, don't
twist; instead, your
shoulders and hips
should face forward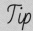

With practice, you
will be able to
squat ever lower

4 Return to your deep squat position,
bending your arms back in front of you.
Focus on getting as low as you can into
the squat, and keep your weight
behind you.

5 Now kick the opposite leg in front.
Repeat, alternating the kicking leg, for
60 seconds. Focus on keeping your
balance and ensuring your hips remain
pointing forwards.

MINUTE 5

Plié squat

This is amazing at targeting and toning your inner thighs, and you can also really work on your abs at the same time. Just remember to keep your belly button pulled in towards your spine throughout the move, and focus on getting as exaggerated a range of motion as possible.

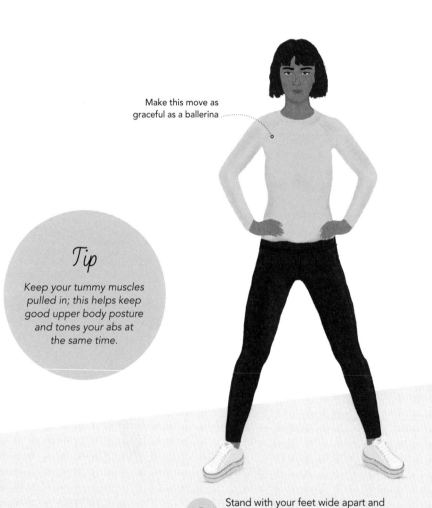

Make this move as graceful as a ballerina

Tip

Keep your tummy muscles pulled in; this helps keep good upper body posture and tones your abs at the same time.

1   Stand with your feet wide apart and your toes pointing out at a 45-degree angle. Place your hands on your hips.

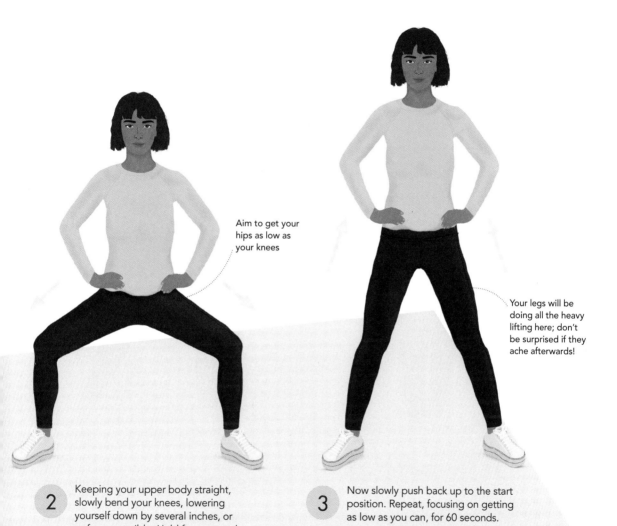

Aim to get your hips as low as your knees

Your legs will be doing all the heavy lifting here; don't be surprised if they ache afterwards!

2 Keeping your upper body straight, slowly bend your knees, lowering yourself down by several inches, or as far as possible. Hold for a second.

3 Now slowly push back up to the start position. Repeat, focusing on getting as low as you can, for 60 seconds.

MINUTE 6

Ballerina circles

If you need to, for balance, you can use a chair for this one. This move is a little lower in intensity than the previous exercise, but don't be fooled, you are still working hard. The circles give you a lovely Transverse (rotational) move through the hips (see p68), so you get to lift and sculpt your lower body.

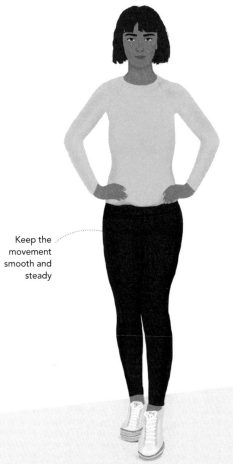

Keep the movement smooth and steady

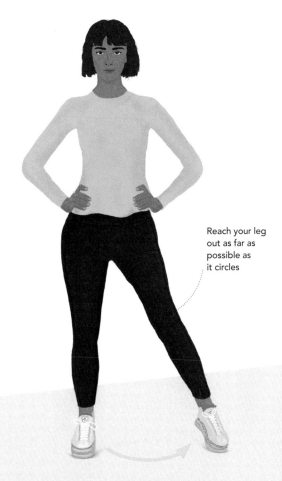

Reach your leg out as far as possible as it circles

1 Standing with good posture, rest your weight on your right leg, with a slightly bent ("soft") right knee, and extend your left foot in front of you. Place your hands on your hips. (Or if you are using a chair, place your right hand on the chair.)

2 Slowly take your left foot out to the front and make a big circle, first to the side, keeping it low to the floor and making the circle as big as you can.

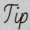

Tip

Imagine that you are drawing a big circle on the ground with your foot.

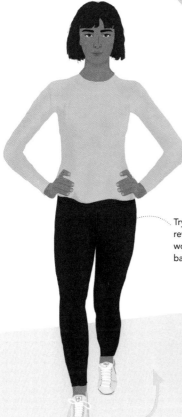

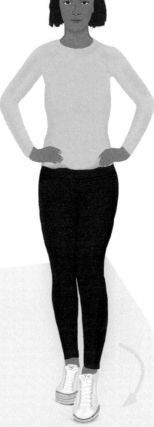

Try to do this in reverse every other workout, to make backwards circles

3 Continue the circle, bringing your left foot behind you as far as you can. Keep your hips facing forward, don't twist them, for the best results.

4 Bring the left foot back to the front, and keep making circles with it for 30 seconds. Then change to making circles with the right foot for the final 30 seconds.

MINUTE 7

Rainbow curtsy

This move is going to help get your heart rate up, so you are burning a high amount of calories. The Frontal (lateral) step behind (see p68) is great for shaping and sculpting your legs. Focus on keeping your balance here; as ever, keeping your tummy muscles pulled in will help to stabilize your core, which in turn will help your balance.

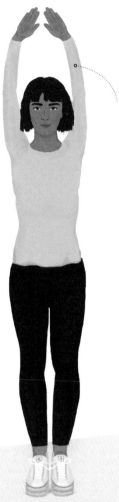

Reach up high so you can feel the stretch in your spine

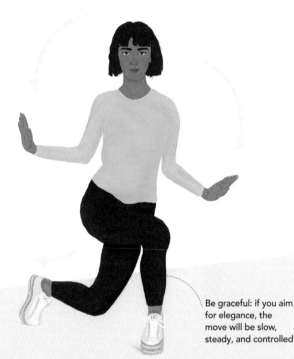

Be graceful: if you aim for elegance, the move will be slow, steady, and controlled

1   Stand with good posture, with both arms directly above your head.

2   Now step one leg back and behind you, as if you are curtsying, and, at the same time, draw both your arms down to your sides, still keeping your upper body straight.

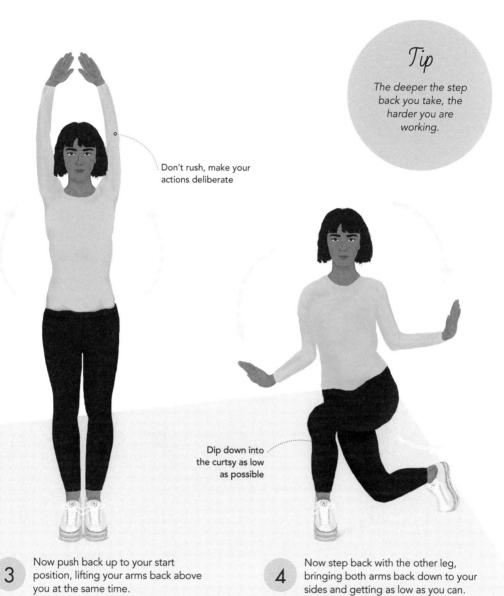

Don't rush, make your actions deliberate

Tip

The deeper the step back you take, the harder you are working.

Dip down into the curtsy as low as possible

3 Now push back up to your start position, lifting your arms back above you at the same time.

4 Now step back with the other leg, bringing both arms back down to your sides and getting as low as you can. Repeat the curtsies, alternating legs, for 60 seconds.

MORE WAYS TO LOVE YOUR LEGS

7 TIPS

1 STEP TO IT.

Walking is a great way to tone and sculpt your legs. Over this 7-day challenge, set yourself another goal of completing a certain amount of steps a day. Nowadays most phones have a step counter, but if yours doesn't, you can pick up pedometers very cheaply and clip them onto your clothing or pop them in a pocket and they will tell you how many steps you have taken. You will be surprised how quickly they add up. So – don't be shocked – but I am going to set you a good challenge here: aim for 8,000–10,000 steps a day. Just do a quick walk in the morning, then a walk around the block at lunchtime, then do some shopping. And, of course, marching on the spot at home or going up and down stairs will make sure you hit that target daily. This will not only help to get your legs in amazing shape but, better still, give you a massive health and fitness boost.

2 LEG SCRUB.

Make your own leg scrub, as a great way to help you get super-silky smooth skin. Let's be honest, anything that makes you feel good is a positive step towards looking and feeling your best.

What you need:
1 tbsp ground coffee
2 tsp sea salt flakes
3 tbsp olive oil

Mix all the ingredients in a bowl. When you're in the shower, apply to your legs, rub in and massage, then rinse off for super-silky skin. This has the bonus of boosting circulation in your legs.

FAQ

I store fat on hips and thighs. What are the best exercises to reduce this?

Our body shape is in our DNA and we should embrace it. Focus on you, don't compare yourself to others, but be the best version of yourself instead. If you want to work your hips and thighs, the Love My Legs workout is great, as well as walking, which is a lovely way to tone and sculpt through the hips. All my workouts help reduce body fat, so you will see great results.

3 TEETH AND TONE.

A fun way to add in little extra ways of toning your legs daily is if you include them in an existing daily ritual. So, from now on, every time you brush your teeth, simply do some calf raises. Stand with your feet hip-width apart, then slowly lift both your heels off the floor, coming up onto your tiptoes, hold, then slowly lower down.

4 TV SQUEEZE.

When you are watching TV, you can quickly do this easy inner thigh-toning squeeze. Sit with good posture on the edge of the sofa, with both feet firmly on the ground. Now place a cushion or pillow between your knees. Squeeze as hard as you can, imagining you are trying to get your knees to touch through the cushion. Hold for several seconds, then slowly release the pressure. Keep doing this several times and you will – for sure – feel and see the results through your thighs.

5 UP AND DOWN.

When you get a spare few moments (and if nobody is looking), try this great lower body exercise. Place a chair against the wall. Now simply sit on it with good posture, then stand up straight, again with good posture, then sit back down. Do as many as you can.

FAQ

I have leg cellulite. Will exercise get rid of it?

There are probably only a handful of adults in the world who are cellulite-free. There are, however, lifestyle factors that help reduce it. Cellulite is – simply put – squished-up fat cells. When we start reducing body fat, it will diminish. Take daily exercise, eat a healthy diet, avoid sugar and processed foods, drink plenty of water, and increase your circulation in the areas where you have cellulite (try my home-made scrub, see left).

6 TAKE TWO.

We have heard it a million times: take the stairs. But I have one better than that for you: take 2 stairs at a time! This puts your body through a deep range of motion, especially your lower body, more like performing a lunge, so it will help you with toning. Plus, you get to the top more quickly!

7 TALK AND TONE.

Next time your best friend phones for a chat, make the most of it. Keep moving as you talk, even just around the house, and avoid sitting down anywhere for the length of the conversation. Imagine how many steps you could get in during a 20-minute call…

7-MINUTE

CARDIO-BOOST & SCULPT SEATED WORKOUT

Just because this workout is seated, don't be fooled into thinking that it's easy. You are going to be investing in your most important muscle of all – your heart – as the moves are great for cardiovascular health. Not only that, but the exercises here will tone and sculpt your body, supercharge your energy levels, and build your confidence.

MEASURE YOUR PROGRESS

For this workout, monitor your improvement by measuring your resting heart rate. As a general rule, a low heart rate shows good cardiovascular fitness. However, it's pointless comparing your results to someone else's; this is about *your* journey. You can use a wearable device, if you have one. Or it's easy to do manually:

HOW TO MEASURE YOUR PULSE
Place your index and middle fingers on your inner wrist and find your pulse. You will need a timer that counts seconds. Time your heart beat for 15 seconds. Make a note of it. Now, multiply the number by four: this is your resting heart rate. Write it on your checklist (see p30).

Take your resting pulse rate before drinking caffeine, as this increases your heart rate. In 7 days, measure it again, at the same time.

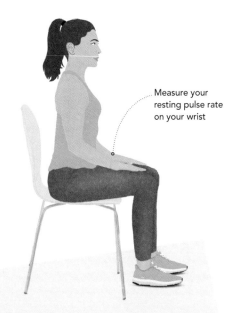

Measure your
resting pulse rate
on your wrist

Tip

If you have a disability, an injury, or wear and tear on your joints, this is the workout for you.

OVERVIEW OF THE WORKOUT

Perform each move, flat out if you can, in the order shown for 1 minute. Don't forget to warm up and cool down (see p20–25).

MINUTE 1	*Run punch*
MINUTE 2	*The ab monster*
MINUTE 3	*Sprint swim*
MINUTE 4	*Power kicks*
MINUTE 5	*Knee crunch & twist*
MINUTE 6	*Thumbs up*
MINUTE 7	*Cupid's arrow*

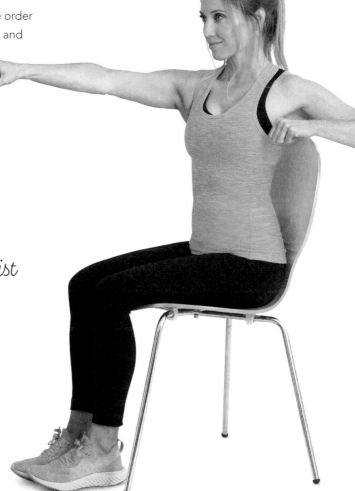

MINUTE 1

Run punch

This exercise really gets your heart rate up and will increase cardiovascular health, as well as toning and sculpting your arms. Whether you're punching or "running", aim to keep each movement as high as possible. I want you to challenge yourself to perform each exercise as fast as you can, too, but keep good posture and ensure your movements are smooth and controlled.

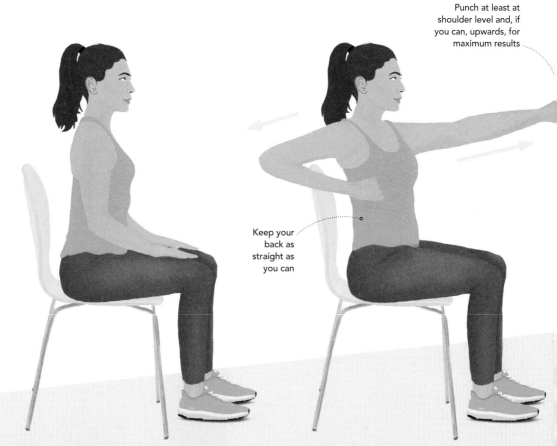

Punch at least at shoulder level and, if you can, upwards, for maximum results

Keep your back as straight as you can

1 Sit with good posture, back straight, shoulders back, and belly button pulled in towards your spine.

2 Now start punching straight out in front, keeping your fists at shoulder level and without dropping the height of your arms. Do this for 10 counts.

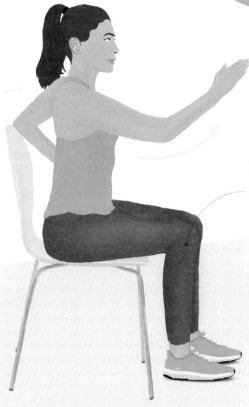

The quicker you can "run", the more effective this will be

3 Now change to "running". Simply mimic the movement your arms would make if you were running: pumping back and forth. Do this for 10 counts. Alternate between punching and "running" for 60 seconds.

MINUTE 2

The ab monster

This one works your abs, as the full rotation engages the oblique muscles that help sculpt your abs, plus the twisting move will help improve your trunk flexibility. I fully expect that you will be able to twist further on day 7 than you could on day 1. As always with my 7-minute workouts, really exaggerating the moves will achieve the best results, and help you get amazing curves in your waist.

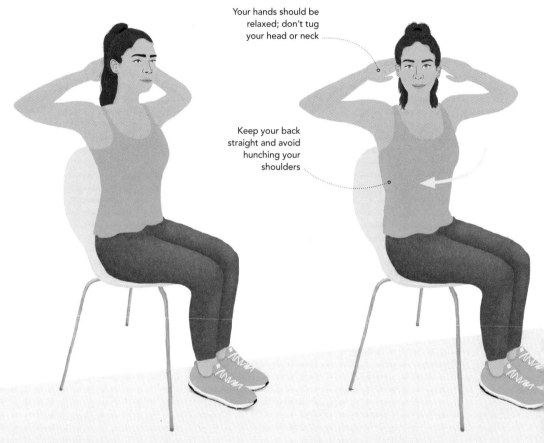

Your hands should be relaxed; don't tug your head or neck

Keep your back straight and avoid hunching your shoulders

1 Sit with good posture, with your feet firmly placed on the ground, hip-width apart. Place your fingertips by the side of your head, with your elbows out to the side, aiming to keep your elbows in line with your shoulders.

2 Now twist to the right from your torso, aiming to take your right elbow out behind you and your left elbow forward. Reach round as far as you can, so you can feel the twist in your waist.

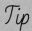

Tip

Keep this move slow and controlled and always aim to twist as far around as you can, so you can feel the exercise working in your waist.

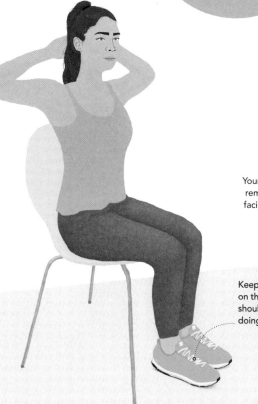

Your hips should remain still, and facing forwards, throughout

Keep your feet flat on the floor, as it should be your waist doing all the work

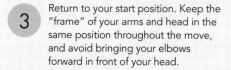

3 Return to your start position. Keep the "frame" of your arms and head in the same position throughout the move, and avoid bringing your elbows forward in front of your head.

4 Twist from your torso once more, this time reaching round to the other side. Continue, alternating side twists, for 60 seconds.

MINUTE 3

Sprint swim

This move – which is just like breaststroke – not only works on toning and sculpting your arms, chest, and upper back, but is also great for your flexibility, as well as for improving your posture. If you can arrange to work out in front of a mirror, it will help you to stop your arms from dropping down; keeping them parallel to the floor will maximize your results.

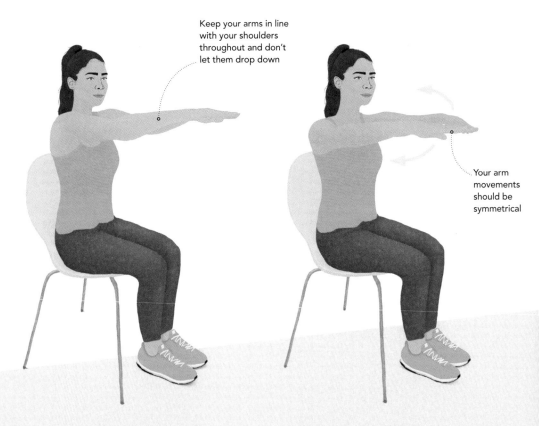

Keep your arms in line with your shoulders throughout and don't let them drop down

Your arm movements should be symmetrical

1 Sit with good posture, with your feet firmly placed on the ground, hip-width apart. Now stretch both arms out directly in front of you at chest height, with your palms facing down.

2 Pull your arms back in an outwards circular motion, drawing back your elbows as if doing breaststroke. Move smoothly and deliberately.

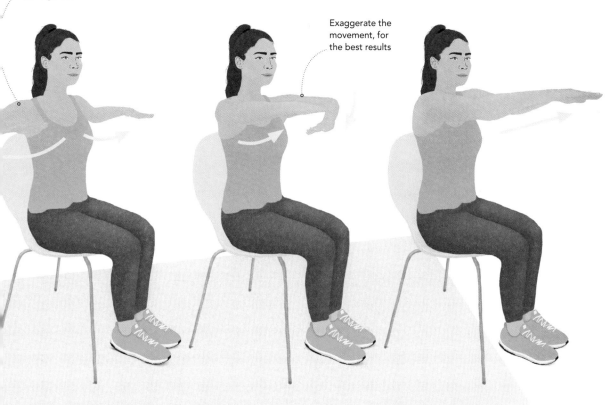

Tip

It is so important to really engage your mind, think of the muscles you are working, and imagine you are swimming in water against a strong current, as this instantly makes your muscles work harder.

Really squeeze your shoulder blades together as your elbows go back

Exaggerate the movement, for the best results

3 Continue the backwards circular motion, taking your elbows slightly behind you.

4 Bring your hands forwards until you can cross them one under the other, close to your body.

5 Now extend both arms back out to the front, palms facing down, as for your start position.

MINUTE 4

Power kicks

This is great for your fitness levels, but it does more than just get you fit. It also sculpts your legs and arms, and even works your core muscles as well. Don't worry if you can't lift your legs as far as in the illustration; don't compare yourself to the picture, just concentrate on lifting your own legs higher every day. And try to punch upwards, for maximum results.

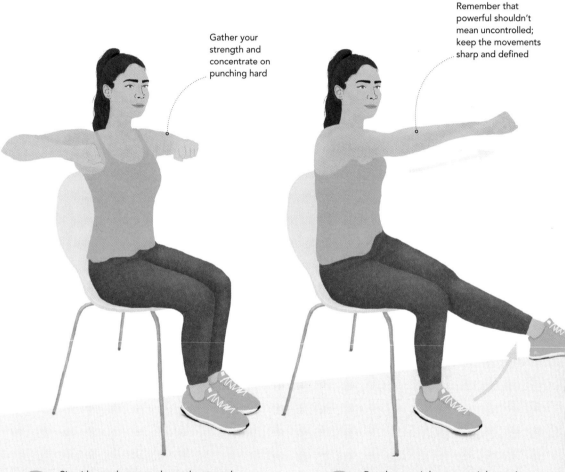

Gather your strength and concentrate on punching hard

Remember that powerful shouldn't mean uncontrolled; keep the movements sharp and defined

1 Sit with good posture, knees bent, and feet flat on the floor. Bend both arms at the elbow and make your hands into fists. Bring your fists up to just in front of your shoulders, elbows behind you.

2 Punch your right arm straight out in front at chest height and – at the same time – kick the opposite leg out, so it is in a straight line from foot to hip. Your left arm should be behind you.

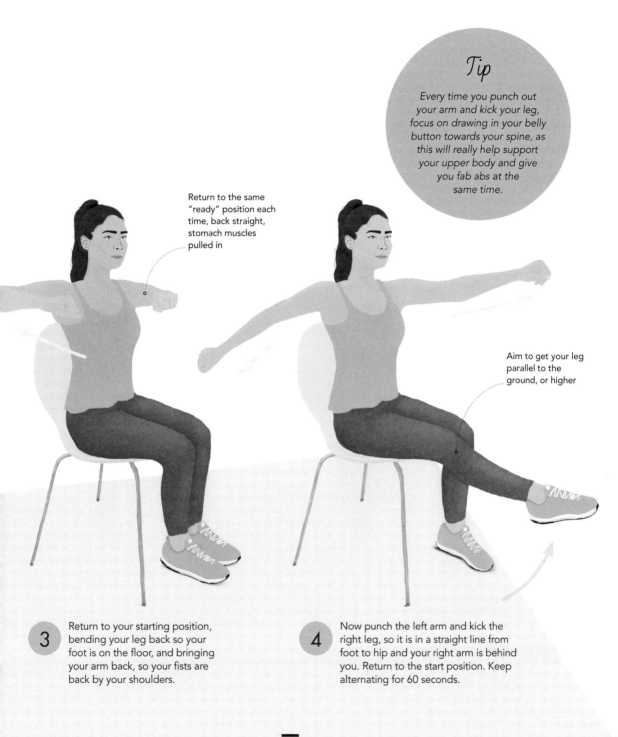

Tip

Every time you punch out your arm and kick your leg, focus on drawing in your belly button towards your spine, as this will really help support your upper body and give you fab abs at the same time.

Return to the same "ready" position each time, back straight, stomach muscles pulled in

Aim to get your leg parallel to the ground, or higher

3 Return to your starting position, bending your leg back so your foot is on the floor, and bringing your arm back, so your fists are back by your shoulders.

4 Now punch the left arm and kick the right leg, so it is in a straight line from foot to hip and your right arm is behind you. Return to the start position. Keep alternating for 60 seconds.

MINUTE 5

Knee crunch & twist

This move engages so many muscles and, by adding the Transverse (rotational) twist (see p68), you work lots of the side muscles that can often be neglected. Plus this exercise will help to keep your heart rate up, so you can ensure you are getting super-fit. Make sure you do not strain your neck; it should remain comfortable throughout.

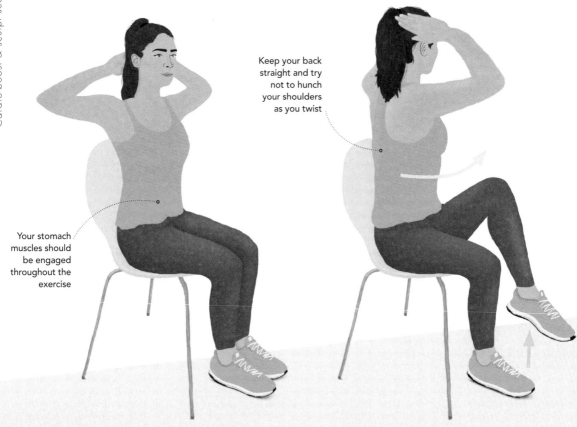

Keep your back straight and try not to hunch your shoulders as you twist

Your stomach muscles should be engaged throughout the exercise

1 Sit nice and tall, with good posture and both feet firmly on the floor, hip-width apart. Bring both arms out to the sides, with your elbows bent and in line with your shoulders, palms facing forwards.

2 Now raise your left foot off the ground, lifting your knee up, and at the same time twist through your torso, aiming to get your right elbow as close to your knee as you can. Hold for a second.

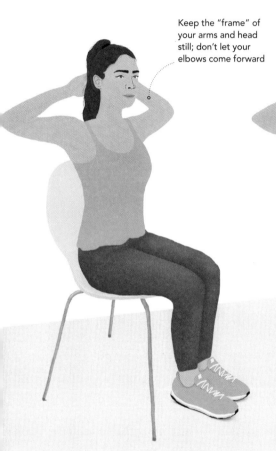

Keep the "frame" of your arms and head still; don't let your elbows come forward

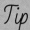

Tip

As you lift your leg up, be sure to pull your belly button in tight towards your spine, as this helps work your abs and it also protects your back.

Make sure your feet touch the floor softly, without stamping

3 Return to the start position, again planting your feet firmly on the floor, and keeping your elbows at the same height as your shoulders.

4 Lift your right foot off the floor, bringing your knee up, and twist through your torso to bring your left elbow towards it. Then return to your start position. Continue for 60 seconds.

MINUTE 6

Thumbs up

This move really helps to reduce any tightness in your chest and is perfect for upper body posture. In step 4, when you take your arms above your head, you up the intensity of the move, so you get a great cardio effect, as your heart has to work harder when your arms are above heart level. This is a great tip to remember: when you can, get those arms in the air!

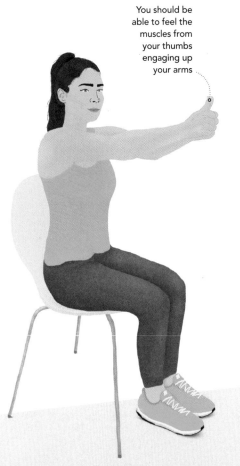

You should be able to feel the muscles from your thumbs engaging up your arms

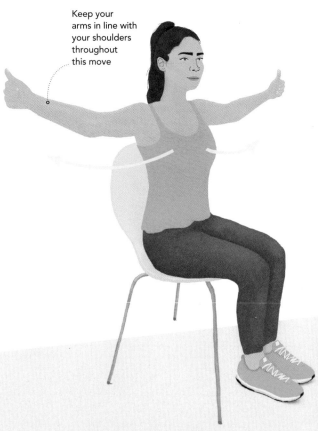

Keep your arms in line with your shoulders throughout this move

1. Sit with good posture, chest lifted, and shoulders pulled back, feet firmly on the floor hip-width distance apart. Extend both arms straight out in front, with your palms facing inwards, and your thumbs pointing up.

2. In a controlled manner, bring both your arms out to either side, so you are lifting and opening through your chest, still keeping them at the same height.

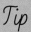

Tip

Perform this in front of the mirror. We all have one stronger side, so one arm may be higher. This is a great time to notice this, and focus on getting your weaker side to the same height.

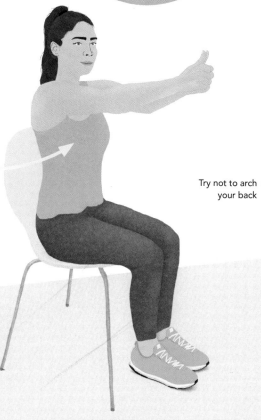

Try not to arch your back

Try to keep right angles at your knees, moving forwards in your chair if necessary

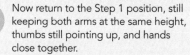

3 Now return to the Step 1 position, still keeping both arms at the same height, thumbs still pointing up, and hands close together.

4 Keeping your hands close to each other, lift both arms directly up above your head. Hold for a second. Continue for 60 seconds.

MINUTE 7

Cupid's arrow

This helps to strengthen and shape through your waist, will enhance your upper body flexibility and mobility, and shape and sculpt through your back and shoulders. Again, you are using Transverse (rotational) moves (see p68), to strengthen your sides and produce some fabulous curves in your waist. As ever, make sure you twist as far as you can, to gain the maximum benefits.

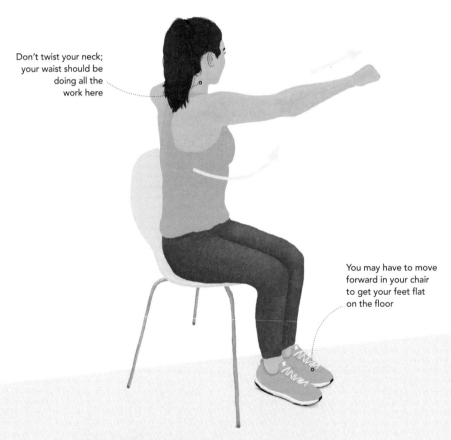

Don't twist your neck; your waist should be doing all the work here

You may have to move forward in your chair to get your feet flat on the floor

1 Sit with good posture, feet flat on the floor and hip-width distance apart. Extend your right arm straight out in front of you, your left arm should be pulled back so your elbow is behind you and your hand is by your shoulder.

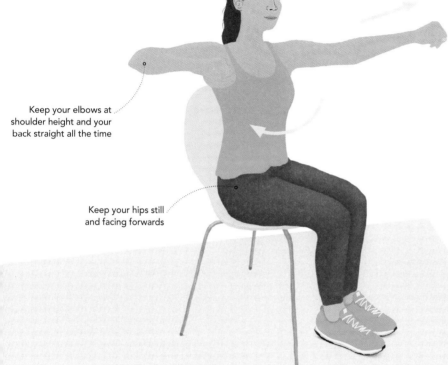

Tip

Keep this movement slow and controlled, and imagine that you are pulling back that bow as far as you can.

Keep your elbows at shoulder height and your back straight all the time

Keep your hips still and facing forwards

2 Now change the arms: pull back the straight arm, and, at the same time, extend the other arm forwards (just like you are shooting a bow and arrow).

Simply keep alternating from one to the other, aiming, as you pull the arm back, to slightly rotate through your torso: you should feel this stretch in your waist. Do this continuously for 60 seconds.

MORE WAYS TO ENHANCE YOUR SEATED WORKOUT

7 TIPS

1 ... AND BREATHE.
Deep breathing enhances many bodily functions – it increases your stamina, and reduces stress and anxiety – and overall, these help with your fitness, too. So try to make it a habit to take time to do some deeper breaths in the morning, noon, and in the evening.

Sit tall and with good posture. Now breathe in through your nose for a count of 3 seconds – or until you feel you have taken a big, deep breath – hold for a couple of seconds, then slowly exhale through your mouth for several seconds, until you have exhaled all your breath. Repeat several times. The more you practise, you will find you can take deeper breaths, hold them for longer, and exhale for longer.

2 SPICE IT UP.
A great tip for your nutrition that is really easy to apply. If you have too much salt in your diet, simply swap it for spices or herbs instead. This is so much better for your cardiovascular health, and also many spices contain plenty of minerals and vitamins.

Here are some good choices:
Allspice
Cayenne pepper
Ginger
Oregano
Thyme

3 BE INSPIRED.
Nothing is more uplifting than real life stories of people overcoming so much. Find an autobiography of someone you admire… or write one. Go to p14 for 7-minute workout success stories!

FAQ

What is the best time of the day to exercise?

Your timeslot has to work for you, to make it part of your lifestyle. The benefit of mornings is that you will take control of your health at the start of the day. In the evenings, the benefit is that you will be more flexible, as your muscles are warmer, and it can also aid sleep. Working out at lunchtime has the benefit of helping to increase your energy levels and curb urges for sugary snacks during the mid-afternoon dip.

4 MASTER YOUR OWN JUICE.

This is really fun. These fruits, vegetables, and seeds are great for your heart and your health. Pick 3–5 of them and create a super-healthy juice, using a maximum of 3 pieces of fruit and as many vegetables as you can.

So make a single combination, or create a new juice for each day of the 7-day challenge. To make, juice vegetables and up to 3 items from this list, adding water if needed, until you have a consistency you like:

Apple
Avocado
Banana
Beetroot (beets)
Berries
Cherries
Chia seeds
Flaxseeds
Kiwi
Orange
Spinach

5 BE YOUR OWN DJ.

Music is a great way to get you in the mood to work out. It can instantly make you feel upbeat and energized. Make a 7-minute workout playlist. Most songs are only 3–4 minutes long, so you only need a handful. Make a different list every week for each of the 7-minute workouts. (Confession: one of my tunes will always be ABBA's "Super Trouper".)

FAQ

Do I need to use weights?

I've found that body weight is super-effective. Think about extending your arm straight out in front – you'll soon feel how heavy it is. Trust me, 60 seconds is a long time, and my exercises start to feel challenging at the 40-second mark, which is great because it is achievable to keep going. This is the magic 20 seconds when we get amazing results, just by using our own body weight. You don't need weights, and you can work out anywhere.

6 ROLL IT AND CLIMB IT.

I'm always trying to come up with new ideas on how to keep fit. Here's one. Roll 2 dice, then make the results into a 2-digit number (a roll of 3 and 6 makes 36.) With your upper body, mimic the move of climbing up 36 rungs of a ladder. (Each time you lift an arm is 1 rung.) You could get up to 66!

7 ICE CUBE .

Imagine someone has just dropped an ice cube down your back. See how you instantly pull back your shoulders and lift your chest? Write the word "ice cube" on a post-it note (or several) and place it (or them) where you often see it. This way, you get a visual prompt to sit with great posture. And the more often you do this, the easier it will be to maintain good form.

7-MINUTE

CALORIE-BURNING WORKOUT

This workout really super-charges your metabolism; you will burn off serious amounts of calories in just 7 minutes, and also raise your calorie burn for hours after. This routine is ideal if you are trying to reach a healthy weight, as it melts off fat fast. It works because not only are all the 7 moves I have selected for you multicompound (they work lots of muscle groups at once), as are all the other routines in this book, but this one also has some "plyometric" (jumping) moves, that need a little more energy. I've been kind and interspaced these with no-jump moves… but those are still big calorie-burners.

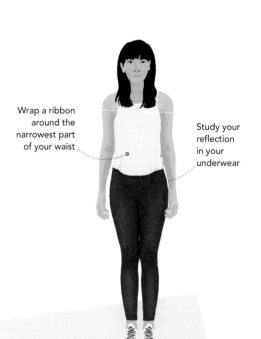

Wrap a ribbon around the narrowest part of your waist

Study your reflection in your underwear

MEASURE YOUR PROGRESS

There are a couple of tests you can do. You can do both or just one, the choice is yours.

METHOD 1 – LOVE MY RIBBON

Wrap a ribbon round your waist. Mark where it meets. After 7 days, it will be shorter.

METHOD 2 – THE MIRROR

Stand in front of the mirror in your underwear. As we tend to lose weight from different areas, it is a good way of assessing weight loss. Take a long look. See how incredible your body is, it gives you life, so start loving it. After 7 days, repeat. If you've stuck to the plan, you'll notice a change.

OVERVIEW OF THE WORKOUT

Perform each move, flat out if you can, in the order shown for 1 minute. Don't forget to warm up and cool down (see p20–25).

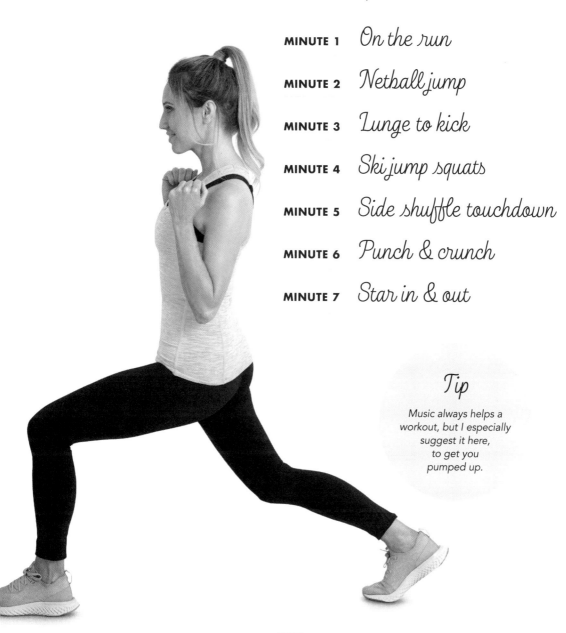

MINUTE 1 *On the run*

MINUTE 2 *Netball jump*

MINUTE 3 *Lunge to kick*

MINUTE 4 *Ski jump squats*

MINUTE 5 *Side shuffle touchdown*

MINUTE 6 *Punch & crunch*

MINUTE 7 *Star in & out*

Tip

Music always helps a workout, but I especially suggest it here, to get you pumped up.

MINUTE 1

On the run

This fast-paced cardio move is a great way to strip off excess body fat and also gives your abs, legs, arms, and rear a great quick toning session at the same time. Try to really exaggerate the movements as you run, as this will give you the best results, and go as fast as you can. Keep it up for the full 60 seconds and your body will thank you for it.

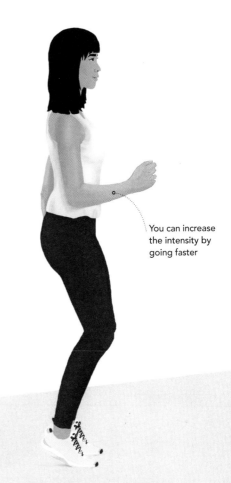

You can increase the intensity by going faster

Tip

If you are a beginner and need this to be a little easier, take it slower, or simply march on the spot and take out the jump.

1 Start by standing with good posture. Engage your abs and glutes, so your body is stabilized, and make sure your knees are soft and not locked. Get ready to run…

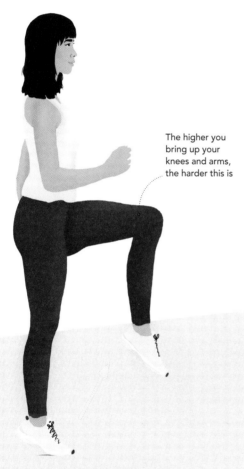

The higher you bring up your knees and arms, the harder this is

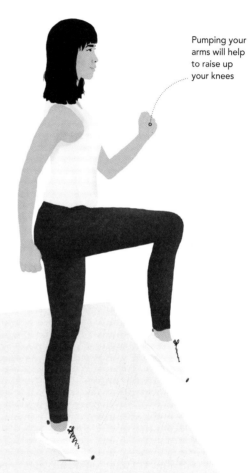

Pumping your arms will help to raise up your knees

2 Now start running on the spot, bringing your left knee and right arm up high as you do so. The higher the better, so aim for your knee to be level with your hip.

3 Alternating from leg to leg, simply imagine you are running fast on the spot, again, always trying to lift your knee as high as possible. Do this for 60 seconds.

MINUTE 2
Netball jump

This Frontal (lateral) travelling move (see p68) with an added Plyometric jump (see p104), targets lots of major muscle groups. Importantly, it works on the muscles on each side of your thighs, as well as your lower body in general, due to the travelling squat. And, at the same time, the jumping is doing wonders for your cardiovascular health.

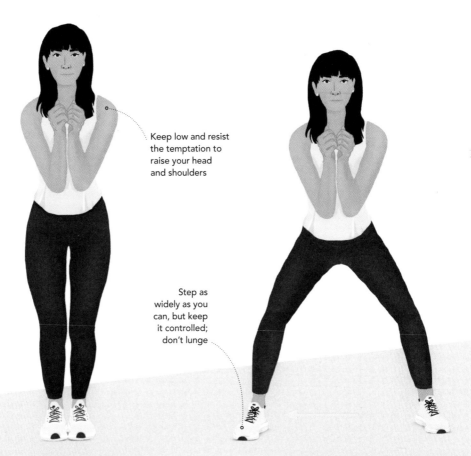

Keep low and resist the temptation to raise your head and shoulders

Step as widely as you can, but keep it controlled; don't lunge

1 Start in a squat position with your elbows and knees bent. Aim to get as low as possible, while engaging your core for optimum balance.

2 Keeping low and pushing off your left foot, take a big deep side step to the right, moving as far as you can. Bring your left foot across to join your right, still staying low.

Tip

The deeper the step and the higher the jump, the bigger the calorie burn for this move.

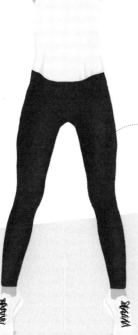

Really put your all into the jump, using your low starting position to add momentum

Engaging your glutes and abs will help to keep the exercise super-effective

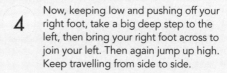

3 Straight away jump up high (imagine you are shooting a goal for netball). Land low, back in your squat position, aiming to keep your balance.

4 Now, keeping low and pushing off your right foot, take a big deep step to the left, then bring your right foot across to join your left. Then again jump up high. Keep travelling from side to side.

MINUTE 3

Lunge to kick

Even though we are not doing any jumping here, this is still a high-intensity move as it is so dynamic (because your body moves from low to high), so will be burning lots of calories. You will find that it is a challenging exercise, but, as with all my moves, the last 20 seconds are where we see the results, so keep going.

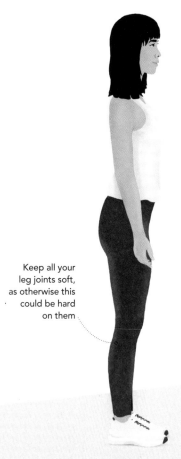

Keep all your leg joints soft, as otherwise this could be hard on them

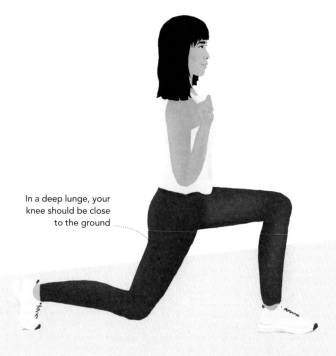

In a deep lunge, your knee should be close to the ground

1 Stand with good posture, feet wider than hip-width apart. You will be challenging your balance throughout this move, so take a moment to stabilize yourself before you begin.

2 Now lunge your right leg behind you; you should have a 90-degree bend in the left leg in front, while the right knee behind should be pointing down to the ground. Your upper body should be straight, arms bent and your hands by your shoulders.

Tip

For balance for this move, it is important to keep your feet wider than hip-width apart, so imagine you are standing with one foot on either side of a railway track.

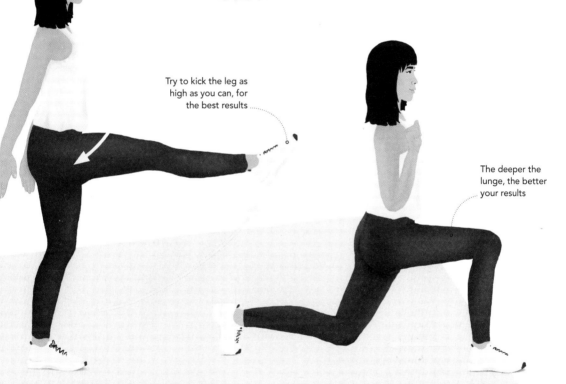

Try to kick the leg as high as you can, for the best results

The deeper the lunge, the better your results

3   Now, driving off your left leg, kick the right leg out in front of you as you come back up to standing. At the same time, your arms should straighten and swing behind you, to aid your balance.

4   Now step the same leg back into the deep lunge and bring your arms back in towards your shoulders. Keep repeating on this leg for 30 seconds, then change to the other leg for the final 30 seconds.

MINUTE 4

Ski jump squats

This travelling Plyometric (jumping) move (see p104) is ticking (checking) so many boxes, it's a serious calorie-burner and a multitoner that will massively boost your fitness. Plus, if you are a skier, this one is amazing at helping to improve your endurance and speed, so use this 7-day workout to get ready for your next skiing trip. This is a multicompound move, working loads of different muscle groups.

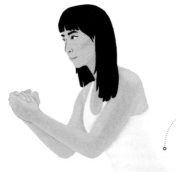

Always keep all your weight behind you when in a squat position

Tip

Make sure, when you land in the squat position, that your knees stay behind the line of your toes.

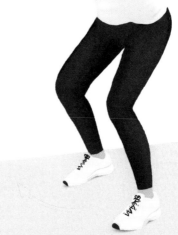

1 Start in a deep squat position with your arms slightly bent and in front of your body. Now jump diagonally in front and to the right, landing in a low squat.

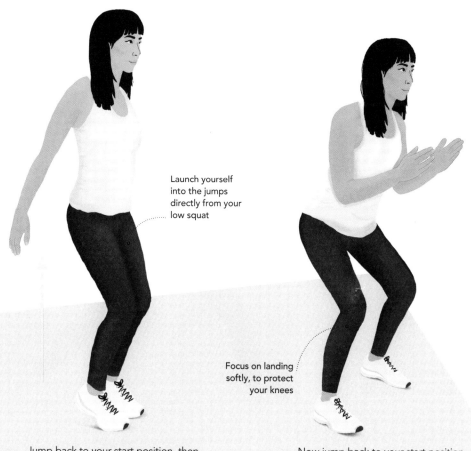

Launch yourself
into the jumps
directly from your
low squat

Focus on landing
softly, to protect
your knees

2   Jump back to your start position, then
straighten up to perform 2 tiny jumps.
Return to the squat and, this time,
jump diagonally in front and to the left,
again landing in a low squat.

3   Now jump back to your start position,
and straighten up to perform 2 tiny
jumps once more. Keep alternating
from side to side for 60 seconds.

MINUTE 5

Side shuffle touchdown

This fast-paced multicompound move works you in a Frontal (lateral) range of motion (see p68), toning up the muscle groups on the sides of your body that often get neglected. At the same time, the dynamic nature of the exercise will be firing up your metabolism, allowing you to burn more calories for hours after the 7 minutes are over.

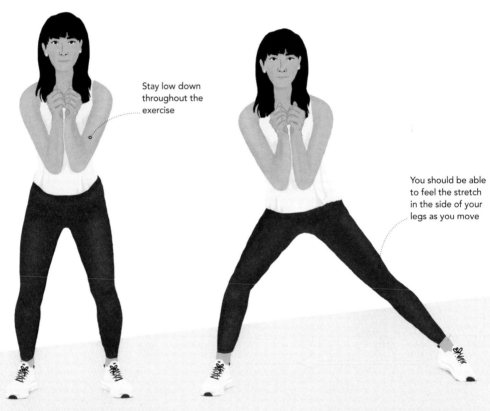

Stay low down throughout the exercise

You should be able to feel the stretch in the side of your legs as you move

1 Start in a deep squat position. Your knees and hips should be bent, and your hands lightly clasped in front.

2 Staying low to the ground and stepping sideways, shuffle a couple of paces to the right side (if your room is long enough, make this more). Bring your feet together between each pace.

The deeper you are in a
squat, the more toned you will
get and the more calories you
will burn, so don't forget to
always keep challenging
yourself.

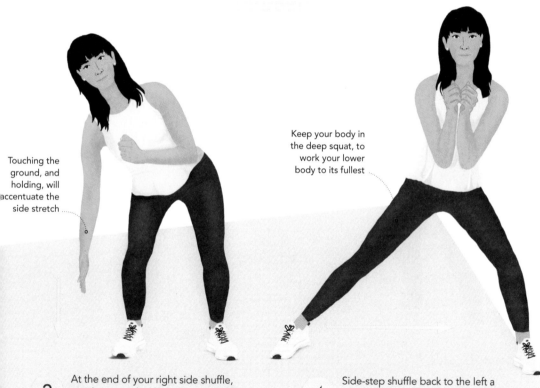

Keep your body in
the deep squat, to
work your lower
body to its fullest

Touching the
ground, and
holding, will
accentuate the
side stretch

3 At the end of your right side shuffle,
tap the ground with the fingertips of
your right hand. Hold your position for
a moment, then return to your squat
position, hands clasped.

4 Side-step shuffle back to the left a
couple of paces, always keeping low,
then touch the ground with your left
fingertips. Continue, alternating sides,
for 60 seconds.

MINUTE 6
Punch & crunch

If you have any stress, this move will get rid of it, as the punching is a great way of relieving stress at the same time as shaping up. I have added a knee crunch, to work even more muscle groups and ensure the whole of your body is exercising hard during this move. You will be performing 4 punches, engaging your arms and chest, then 4 crunches, recruiting the muscles from your glutes and legs.

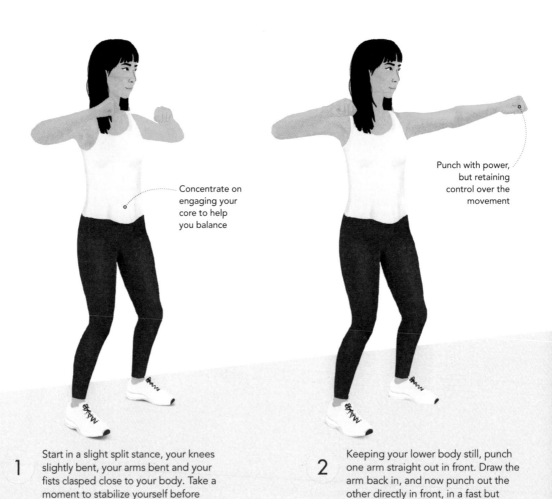

Concentrate on engaging your core to help you balance

Punch with power, but retaining control over the movement

1 Start in a slight split stance, your knees slightly bent, your arms bent and your fists clasped close to your body. Take a moment to stabilize yourself before you begin.

2 Keeping your lower body still, punch one arm straight out in front. Draw the arm back in, and now punch out the other directly in front, in a fast but controlled style. Repeat, so you do 4 punches

Tip

Keep your tummy muscles pulled in tight as you punch and perform the knee lift. This helps protect your back and gives your abs a great toning workout at the same time.

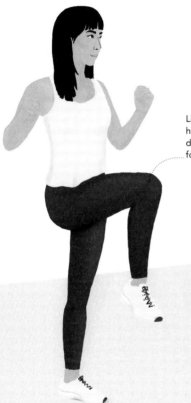

Lift your knee as high as you can during the crunch, for the best results

Always punch up, if possible, or parallel to the ground, but no lower

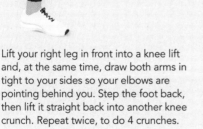

3 Lift your right leg in front into a knee lift and, at the same time, draw both arms in tight to your sides so your elbows are pointing behind you. Step the foot back, then lift it straight back into another knee crunch. Repeat twice, to do 4 crunches.

4 Step the foot back to return to your split stance and repeat Step 2's move of 4 straight punches. Follow this with another 4 knee crunches. Keep repeating this for 30 seconds, then change to the other leg for the final 30 seconds.

MINUTE 7
Star in & out

This move has a little extra twist as, with a traditional star jump, you just bring your arms above your head. I wanted to tweak the star and make sure you use lots more muscles… which, of course, means a high calorie burn.

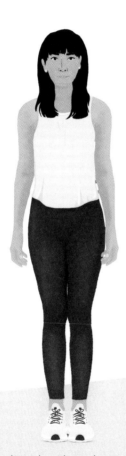

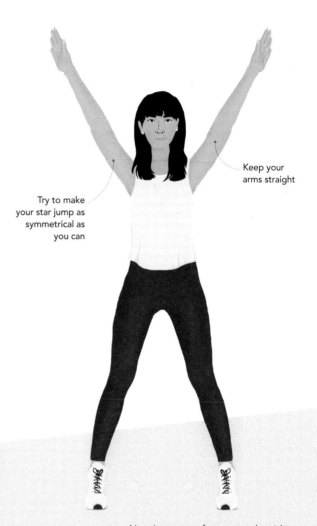

Keep your arms straight

Try to make your star jump as symmetrical as you can

1 Stand upright with good posture, your arms by your sides and your knees soft. Engage your glutes and abs, to aid stabilization, and keep them "switched on" throughout the move.

2 Now jump your feet out to the sides and, at the same time, lift your arms above your head, forming a star jump. Then land back in your start position, keeping the landing soft.

Precision here will bring maximum benefits, so stay controlled

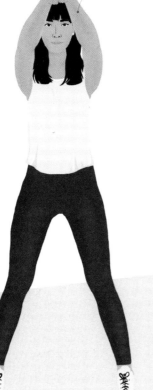

Tip

When you jump, always try to land as softly as you can, to help reduce excessive impact on your joints.

Keep up the intensity and speed right to the end of the 60 seconds

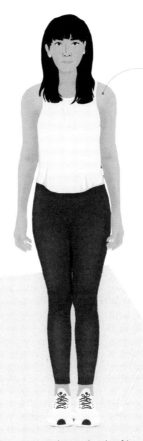

3 This time, repeat the foot movements, jumping them out to the sides, but this time bring your arms up to shoulder height in front of you, palms facing the floor. Land back in your start position.

4 Remember to land softly each time. Keep alternating the arm movements from above your head to out in front, continuously, for 60 seconds.

BURN MORE CALORIES EVERY DAY

7 TIPS

1 TWEAK TO TASTE.

Every little bit helps, so here is a way to burn many more calories easily (each is a minimal amount, but it adds up). These spices all increase your basal metabolic rate, plus they are all loaded with minerals that your body needs, so it's also a great way to boost your nutrition while burning more calories. So here are a few effective spices and a suggestion of what to add them to:

SPICE	ADD TO
Pinch of ground cinnamon	Porridge (oatmeal)
Sprinkle of mustard seeds	Salad
Sprinkle of chilli flakes	Omelette
Pinch of ground turmeric	Latte
Pinch of ground ginger	Smoothie

FAQ

How can I prevent muscle ache after a workout?

Don't be alarmed if you feel stiff the day after doing one of my workouts, as my moves target muscles that often get neglected; aching is good as it means you are toning all over. To help reduce soreness, do my cool down stretches (see p22–25). After that, try a gentle walk; a great way to stretch your muscles. Later in the day, opt for a hot bath or shower, to stimulate blood flow and reduce tension. Ensure you are fully hydrated and focus on performing all my exercises with good posture.

2 PRETEND YOU'RE LATE.

Every time you are walking, even if it is around the house or the supermarket, just go a little faster. On average we walk at a strolling pace, so instead just imagine you are late and step that little bit faster. This can quickly burn extra calories throughout the day, so while you are doing this 7-day challenge, just remember to keep walking everywhere thinking you are late… don't get stressed out by it, though!

3 BAN THE LIFT.

Over the next 7 days, you're taking the stairs. This is a great calorie-burning habit to get into (especially if you take 2 at a time, see p85).

4 SWITCH THE SANDWICH.

Swap your normal sandwich for my breadless version (see p175). You are still getting that easy-to-eat lunch rolled up with your favourite filling, but without the bread. Let me stress that bread is not the enemy, just always go for a healthy version; I think sourdough is the best (see p167). My recipe is just a fun alternative to bread and, of course, contains far fewer calories, so if you tend to eat a sandwich for lunch, this will definitely cut back your calories over the next 7 days.

5 TRY CAULI RICE.

Cauliflower is super-low carb and super-low calorie, and within minutes you can turn it into rice by simply finely grating the florets, or, if you have a blender, pulse it up in there. You can eat it cold and raw, add it to a salad, or, if you want to heat it, microwave cauliflower rice in a covered heatproof bowl for a couple of minutes on High. Swapping rice for cauliflower will save you lots of calories and give you extra vitamins, such as C and K.

6 ARE YOU OR AREN'T YOU?

Let's focus on the hunger question for the next 7 days. If you eat when you're not hungry, that right there is a quick way to gain weight. Sometimes we eat because we are stressed, bored, or emotional, so try to be more mindful over the next 7 days. Obviously, keep eating when you are hungry, just be aware of what is true hunger and what is not. After lunch, when you are about to go for a sweet treat with your tea, ask yourself: are you really that hungry and does your body need it? Try this mindfulness practice around food for 7 days, because if you do normally go for that sugary treat, cutting back on it will make an automatic reduction in your weekly calorie load.

7 BE A FIDGET.

Under the desk at work, tap away, because tapping your feet is moving your body and – as we know – the more we move our body, the more calories we burn. So keep fidgeting.

FAQ

Could I do more than one workout a day?

A 7-minute workout once a day is good enough to get you in shape, increase your health, fitness, wellbeing, and energy levels. Yet often people find, once they have worked out, they have bundles of energy throughout the day, so, obviously, if you fancy doing another, go for it. Our bodies are designed to move and you can squeeze a workout into your lunch hour – or the evening – as they are so short. Listen to your body and do what feels right for you.

7–MINUTE

LITTLE BLACK DRESS WORKOUT

This workout is about toning you up all over and focusing on the key areas that are going to help you look and feel super-confident in your favourite little black dress (LBD). I am going to get you doing some multitasking moves, so you are always toning at least 2 areas for every exercise. This makes it time-friendly, plus each of the moves is a high calorie-burner. I have it all covered for you: we are going to sculpt your shoulders, lift your bottom, give your waist some curves, tone up your thighs, shape your arms, and tighten your tummy!

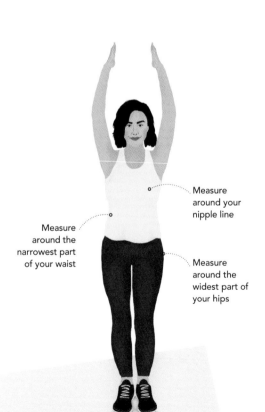

Measure around your nipple line

Measure around the narrowest part of your waist

Measure around the widest part of your hips

MEASURE YOUR PROGRESS
There are a couple of tests you can do. You can do both or just one, the choice is yours.

METHOD 1 – INCH LOSS RESULTS
Measure 3 areas: BUST (around your nipple line); WAIST (the narrowest part); HIPS (the widest part). Record on day 1, then on day 7.

METHOD 2 – FEEL GOOD DRESS FACTOR
On day 1 of the workout, put on your LBD and note the category below that applies best. Do it again on day 7: let's aim for box 3!

	DAY 1	DAY 7
1 – Tight all over, hard to do up		
2 – Feels a little snug		
3 – Amazing. Can't wait to wear it		

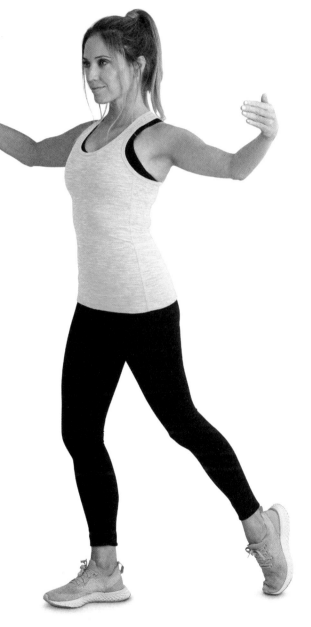

Tip

This workout is targeting your whole body, so get ready to work everything! These full-body moves will really test your balance; aim for controlled, deliberate, and elegant moves, for the best results.

OVERVIEW OF THE WORKOUT

Perform each move, flat out if you can, in the order shown for 1 minute. Don't forget to warm up and cool down (see p20–25).

MINUTE 1 *Shoulder sculpt & bottom lift*

MINUTE 2 *Charleston kicks*

MINUTE 3 *Cardio waist sculptor*

MINUTE 4 *Dream thigh lunge*

MINUTE 5 *Lunge pull downs*

MINUTE 6 *The glute doctor*

MINUTE 7 *Thigh trimmer*

MINUTE 1

Shoulder sculpt & bottom lift

This exercise really gives a great lift to your rear, helping to smooth away bumps and give a streamlined, curvy outline. If you don't like squats, but want to tone your lower body, then this is the move for you – you will love it. Plus, this cardio-boosting exercise will give you some beautiful muscle definition through your shoulders.

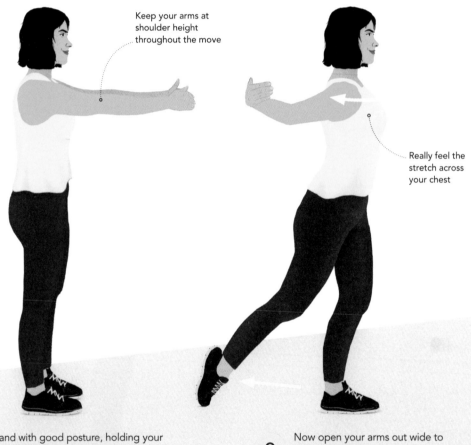

Keep your arms at shoulder height throughout the move

Really feel the stretch across your chest

1 Stand with good posture, holding your arms in front of you with your palms together. Your forearms should be parallel to the floor. Keep your knees slightly bent, to protect the joints.

2 Now open your arms out wide to either side and, at the same time, step one foot directly behind you, while keeping your upper body straight and your hips facing forwards.

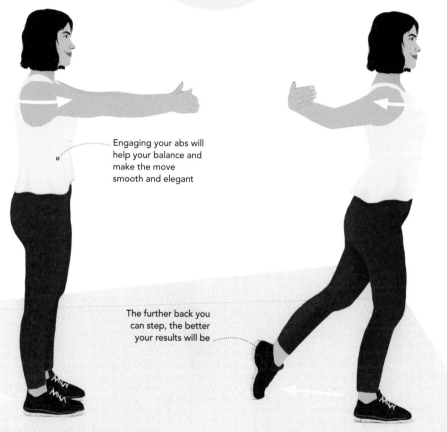

Engaging your abs will help your balance and make the move smooth and elegant

The further back you can step, the better your results will be

3 Bring the foot back to your start position and, at the same time, bring the arms back to the front as if you are clapping, keeping them in line with your shoulders.

4 Repeat the move, but this time take the opposite foot behind. Keep alternating for 60 seconds.

MINUTE 2
Charleston kicks

This move is amazing for sculpting your lower body, especially for toning through your thighs and backside with every kick and jump back. In addition, it is great for balance and flexibility. So even though it is hard, it is so worth it. You may have to practise this once or twice before you nail it and that's normal, so don't worry about it.

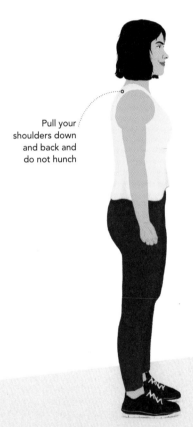

Pull your shoulders down and back and do not hunch

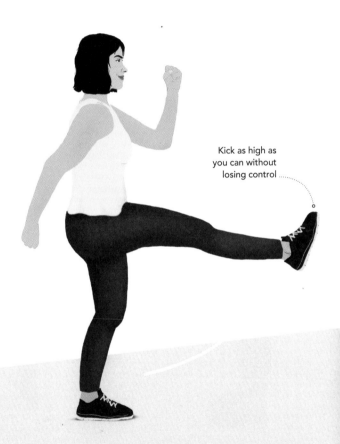

Kick as high as you can without losing control

1 Stand with good posture, with your feet hip-width apart, arms relaxed by your sides, and knee joints soft. Keep those glutes and stomach muscles pulled in tight, to aid your balance.

2 Kick your right leg in front and bring your left arm forward with the kicking leg, bending it slightly; the right arm should swing backwards.

The rear arm helps to balance, so extend it further if needed

Get your leg back as far as you can, so your body goes through its maximum range of movement

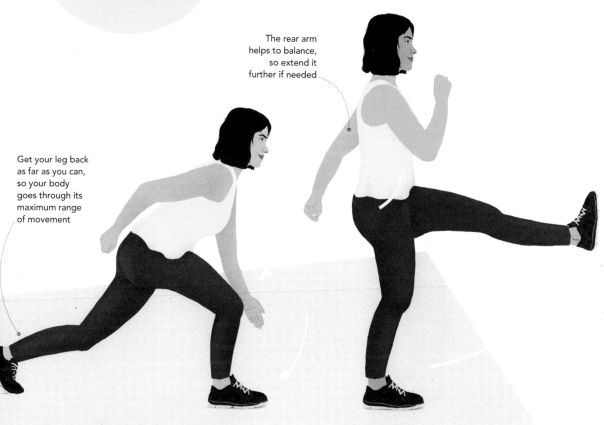

3 Jump the right leg back, transferring your weight to it. At the same time, take your left leg back deep behind you and aim to get the fingers of your left arm close to the floor.

4 Jump straight back up into a kick again, this time with your left leg, with the right arm coming forward and your upper body lifted. Swing the left leg down and transfer your weight to it, then repeat from Step 2, alternating legs, for 60 seconds.

MINUTE 3

Cardio waist sculptor

The Transverse (rotational) twist (see p68) here has you working those internal corset-like oblique muscles to the full, which makes this move amazing at creating lovely curves in your waist. Adding the knee lifts takes the body through a large range of motion, so you are burning off calories at the same time as giving your legs a quick workout.

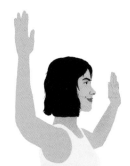

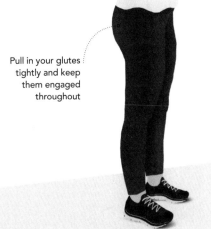

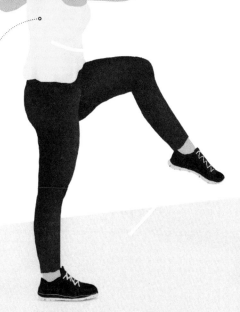

Keep your back straight as you twist, don't hunch your shoulders

Pull in your glutes tightly and keep them engaged throughout

1 Stand with your feet slight wider than hip-width apart, knees slightly bent. Your arms should be bent to a 90-degree angle at the elbow and lifted out to your sides, and your elbows in line with your shoulders.

2 Lift one foot off the floor, bending the leg and aiming to get your knee in line with your hip. At the same time, twist your upper body, aiming to take your opposite elbow towards your knee. Twist far enough around so you can feel it in your waist.

Tip

Keep this move slow and
controlled and really be sure
to work through your fullest
range of motion as you
twist through your
upper body.

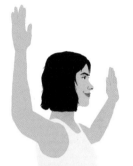

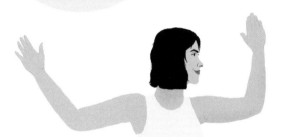

Keep the movement
controlled as you
twist and lift

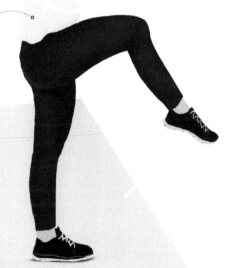

Be sure to land
the foot softly;
don't stamp

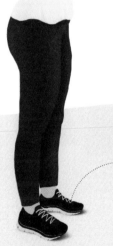

3   Bring the foot back down to the floor
and return your upper body back to
the centre, still keeping your arms
lifted and at a 90-degree angle.

4   Now lift the opposite foot off the floor,
bending the leg and aiming to get
your knee at hip height, then twist your
upper body to bring the opposite
elbow towards your knee.

MINUTE 4

Dream thigh lunge

A sideways lunge is so good for your thighs, as it works through the Frontal (lateral) range of motion (see p68), which tones the muscles down the sides of your legs. You will feel it working instantly. By adding the windmill-like motion of the arms, you are sculpting your upper body at the same time, adding definition to your upper arms and shoulders.

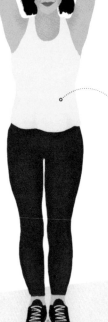

Engage your abs and glutes, and keep those knees soft

Challenge yourself: how low can you go?

1 Stand with good posture, both your arms extended directly above your head, and palms facing in.

2 Step your right leg out deep to the side, and, bending deep from the left knee, going as low as you can, aim to get your right hand close to your left foot. Your other arm should be pointing straight up in the air.

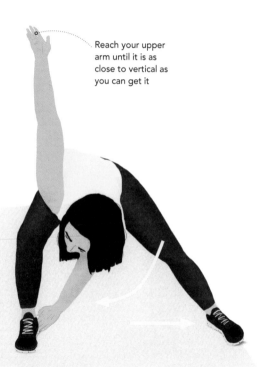

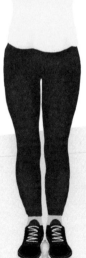

Reach your upper arm until it is as close to vertical as you can get it

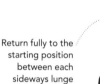

Return fully to the starting position between each sideways lunge

3 Push off from your bent leg, coming back up to standing and taking both arms back to directly above your head, palms facing in.

4 Repeat the move on the same leg for 30 seconds, then change leg for the final 30 seconds.

MINUTE 5

Lunge pull downs

A seemingly simple move, but this one does so much. The reaching up, then pulling down, tones your arms and shoulders. Your abs get a workout to help keep you balanced. And, of course, those glutes and thighs are working overtime to get you into that backward lunge. I mean, that is some serious multitasking...

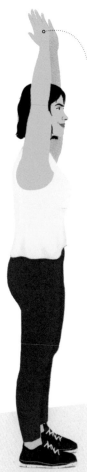

Don't just stand straight, really reach up to the ceiling

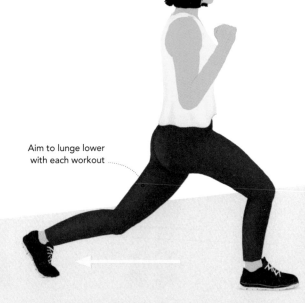

Aim to lunge lower with each workout

1 Stand with your feet shoulder-width apart, both arms directly above your head, palms facing in.

2 Now step one leg behind you to come into a deep lunge position. The knee in front should be bent and the knee behind should be pointing down towards the ground. At the same time, pull both arms down, so your hands end up close by your shoulders with your elbows by your sides.

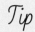

Tip

A backward lunge puts less pressure on your knees than a regular lunge.

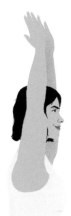

Stay controlled and try not to wobble; engaging your glutes and abs will help

Keep your upper body lifted, don't hunch your shoulders

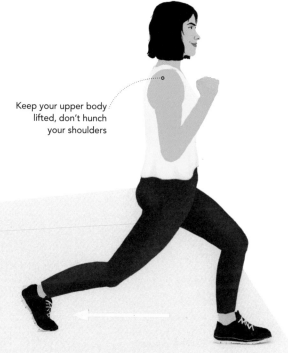

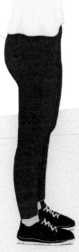

3 Now bring the rear leg back to your start position, lifting your arms back up to their start position, too.

4 Now repeat the move, this time stepping the opposite foot behind into that backward lunge. Keep alternating from leg to leg for 60 seconds.

MINUTE 6

The glute doctor

A great exercise for lifting your glutes and working your abs at the same time, as you engage those muscles for stabilization. If your balance isn't great just yet, help yourself out by using my Tip (see right). However, even if you do use a piece of furniture for support, keep those core muscles pulled in tight!

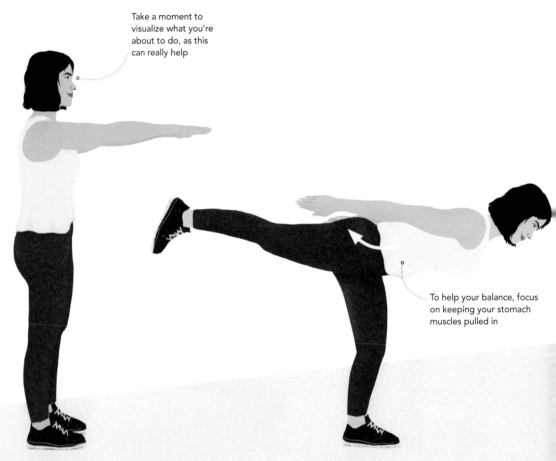

Take a moment to visualize what you're about to do, as this can really help

To help your balance, focus on keeping your stomach muscles pulled in

1 Stand with good posture, with your feet hip-width apart, both arms out directly in front of you, palms facing down.

2 Lift one foot off the floor and behind you, tilting forwards from your hips, and at the same time opening your arms out to the sides. Aim to get your body in a straight line, so the heel on your lifted leg is in line with your head.

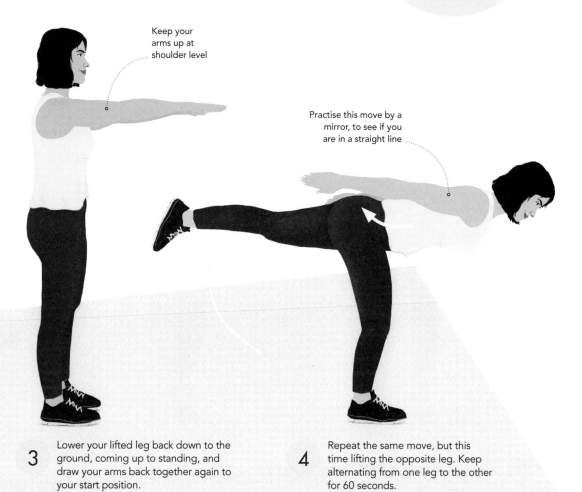

Keep your arms up at shoulder level

Practise this move by a mirror, to see if you are in a straight line

3 Lower your lifted leg back down to the ground, coming up to standing, and draw your arms back together again to your start position.

4 Repeat the same move, but this time lifting the opposite leg. Keep alternating from one leg to the other for 60 seconds.

MINUTE 7

Thigh trimmer

The reason this exercise is great for your thighs is, again, it takes you through that Frontal (lateral) range of motion (see p68), working on the muscles at the side of your legs. And also you work those abs, as you are naturally engaging them to help you with balance and stabilization. The key here is to keep the "frame" of your head, shoulders, and arms static throughout, only moving your legs.

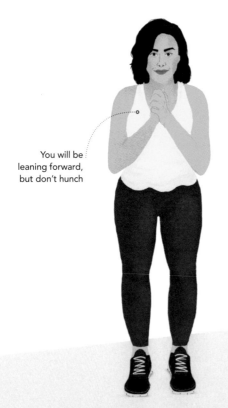

You will be leaning forward, but don't hunch

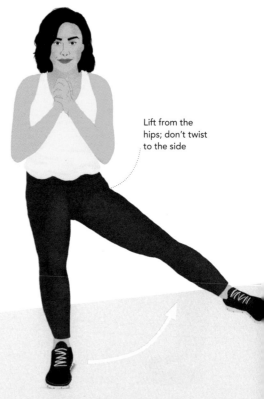

Lift from the hips; don't twist to the side

1 Stand with your feet hip-width apart and have a slight bend in your knees. Your arms should be bent and your hands lightly clasped together in front of you.

2 Now lift one leg off the floor and out to the side, still keeping your body – and especially your hips – facing forwards.

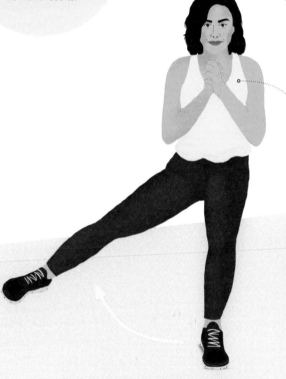

Remember to keep your upper body still; only move your legs

3 Step the foot back down, then immediately lift the other leg off the floor. Keep alternating from one leg to the other for 60 seconds.

GET THE MOST FROM THE LBD WORKOUT

7 TIPS

1 PLAN AHEAD.

The expression "if you fail to plan, you plan to fail" is so true. If you really want to succeed in healthy weight management, then planning meals in advance is an absolute winner. I swear, this really works. Making healthy food choices not only gets you looking great, but will be a great health boost. First, simply go to page 158 for 35 delicious healthy choices to take you from dawn to dusk. Now, write out your 3 meals a day, plus snack, for the next 7 days. Follow it. That's all!

Q&A

What is the best way to keep fit?

Make it a habit, part of your life. This is why my 7-minute workouts are so popular and help literally millions of people worldwide, because they are so do-able, quick, easy to follow, and effective. You can do them wherever you are. And, when you are fit, you have the energy to keep going. Before you know it, they are part of your life. In my professional opinion, a quick home workout is the best option.

2 ORDER SMALL.

Please note: it is so important to always stay within a healthy weight range. I would never advise anyone to lose weight if they don't need to. However, this is a quick and easy way to lose a couple of inches, so if you have a big event coming up and want to be feeling great and super-confident in your favourite outfit, just stick with smaller portions. If you look at dinner plates from the 1970s, they look like our side plates today. Everything we get served or buy now is nearly double what it was years ago, which doesn't help – a double portion means double calories; for example:

Large latte is about 186 calories
Small latte is about 84 calories

3 BE ACCOUNTABLE.

Why not get a friend to take part in this 7-day challenge with you, so you are accountable to each other and you can work out together, no matter where you are in the world. Just Facetime each other and get the book ready in front of you… it's a fun way to work out, then you can catch up afterwards.

4 MANAGE YOUR STRESS.

Stress can increase stomach fat. When we are stressed, we produce higher levels of cortisol, which stores tummy fat. So take time out and try and put yourself under less stress. The next time you feel stressed, do some exercise: it could be just a minute jogging on the spot, but it will help prevent you from storing body fat caused by stress.

5 VISUALIZE YOU IN THAT DRESS.

As our goal is about you looking and feeling your best, use visualization, as your mind controls your body and actions. Every morning when you wake up, picture how fabulous you are going to look in that dress, and know that by doing your workout that day, you are going to achieve that. If you encounter an obstacle during the day that may prevent you working out, or making healthy food choices, simply picture how you want to look in that dress.

6 GO SLOW.

This is a good habit to get into and it is so simple. Chew slowly and be mindful of every mouthful. Instead of eating quickly at your desk, or rushing through your lunch, take it slow. This can help increase levels of appetite-suppressing hormones, and prevent you overeating when you are not actually hungry.

Q&A

Is it important to track your calories?

Over my years helping people with successful weight loss and maintainance, I've found that "calorie-aware" is better than "calorie-obsessed". I encourage clients to learn how to be their healthiest, not their skinniest. Think of the food you eat a lot: be aware of its calories, but don't obsess. Life is about balance; don't put yourself under a regimen in which you are measuring out exact amounts. And, of course, choose healthy, fresh, natural foods.

7 DANCE LIKE NOBODY IS WATCHING.

OK, so this one is fun. If you want to give your body a quick workout, then draw your curtains, put on your favourite song, and dance like nobody is watching. Dancing is a great way to increase your energy levels, burn some calories, and tone up all over, plus you can practise your dance moves for when you are wearing your little black dress at the end of this 7-day challenge! In addition, it will lift your mood, and positivity is so important when you are challenging yourself.

7-MINUTE

SUPER-HEALTH-FIX WORKOUT

This 7-minute workout is going to give your health and fitness the ultimate makeover. We are going to focus on lots of different components of your health: endurance, balance, flexibility, and strength. The 7 minutes you put in every day over the next 7 days will be investing in your health; the best investment you'll ever make. So, for this routine, we are actually going to use a prop (a first for this book)! Don't worry, you don't need to buy anything, it's just a cushion or a pillow. You will love this fun workout and you'll be amazed at the effect that using the pillow has on your balance and stability.

MEASURE YOUR PROGRESS

Test your cardiovascular fitness with this very simple exercise.

Find a safe route that is a loop, exactly 1 mile (1.6km) long from your door. (Use online maps to help you to find one.) Now complete the distance in your fastest time. That's it. You can run, walk or jog, or a mixture of all 3, just aim for your best time.

Then after you have completed your 7-day challenge, complete the same route and see if you can beat the time. If you have stuck to the challenge, I know you will knock seconds off it.

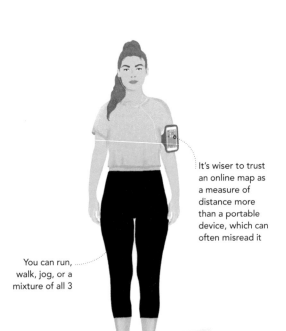

It's wiser to trust an online map as a measure of distance more than a portable device, which can often misread it

You can run, walk, jog, or a mixture of all 3

	TIME
BEFORE	
AFTER	
IMPROVED BY	

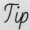
OVERVIEW OF THE WORKOUT

Perform each move, flat out if you can, in the order shown for 1 minute. Don't forget to warm up and cool down (see p20–25).

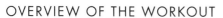

MINUTE 1   *Give me 10*

MINUTE 2   *The steady squat*

MINUTE 3   *Under-knee pass*

MINUTE 4   *Touch down*

MINUTE 5   *Stability punch*

MINUTE 6   *Lunge & twist*

MINUTE 7   *HIIT knee crunch*

MINUTE 1

Give me 10

This is a fun exercise that is great for your endurance, your coordination, and your core. The faster you can run on the spot, the more of a cardio workout you will get. With this first move in the sequence, we are getting used to manipulating a soft item... it's harder than you think! If you prefer a low-impact workout, simply march, rather than jog.

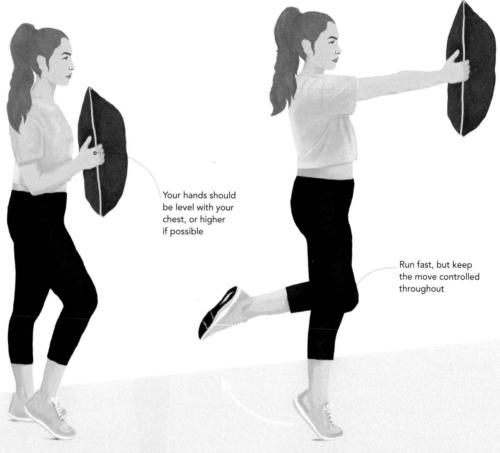

Your hands should be level with your chest, or higher if possible

Run fast, but keep the move controlled throughout

1 Hold on to a cushion at chest height. Stand with good posture, with soft knees. Pull in your glutes and your stomach muscles, to help with your balance and give them a workout, too.

2 Start jogging on the spot and, at the same time, push the cushion out in front of you for a beat, reaching out as far as possible.

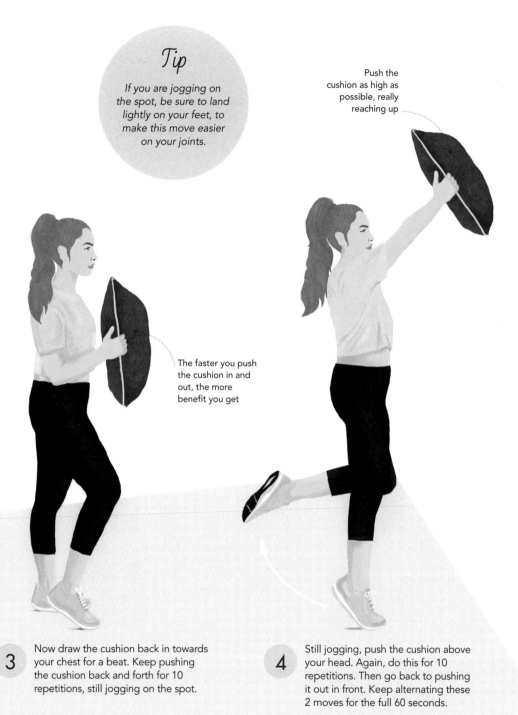

Tip

If you are jogging on the spot, be sure to land lightly on your feet, to make this move easier on your joints.

Push the cushion as high as possible, really reaching up

The faster you push the cushion in and out, the more benefit you get

3 Now draw the cushion back in towards your chest for a beat. Keep pushing the cushion back and forth for 10 repetitions, still jogging on the spot.

4 Still jogging, push the cushion above your head. Again, do this for 10 repetitions. Then go back to pushing it out in front. Keep alternating these 2 moves for the full 60 seconds.

MINUTE 2

The steady squat

With this squat, we are taking working with the cushion to another level. This exercise is great for helping improve stability and balance, as the cushion will be working against those. While you work to keep your balance, you get to engage a few extra stabilizing muscles, too, as standing on the cushion naturally recruits the extra muscles to work.

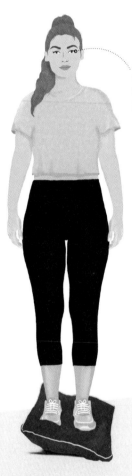

Get your balance before you begin; staring at a fixed point can help

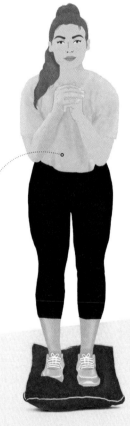

You will notice you need to engage those core muscles for balance

1 Stand on the centre of a cushion, with your feet hip-width apart and with good posture, arms by your sides. Take a moment to get used to the sensation of your unstable base.

2 Bend your knees and come into a low, narrow squat, bringing your arms forwards in front of you at the same time, elbows slightly bent.

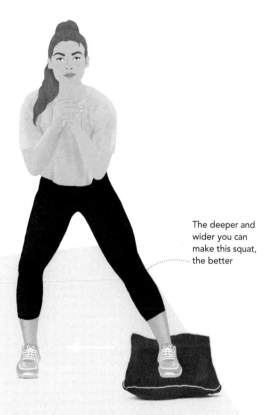

Tip

Do this move in a slow and controlled manner, and remember, when you squat, not to let the line of your knees shoot over your toes, so your weight is always behind you.

Stand tall between squats; don't be tempted to hunch or lean over

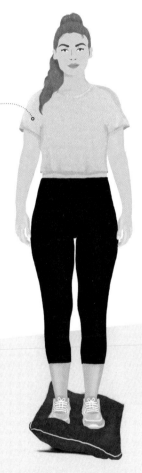

The deeper and wider you can make this squat, the better

3 Come back up to your initial standing position, with your arms by your sides. It is very important to keep your balance – try not to lurch.

4 Now squat again, this time stepping one foot off the cushion so you are in a wide deep squat, bringing your arms forward. Return to standing, arms by your sides. Repeat, first simply squatting, then squatting and stepping off the cushion, alternating legs, for 60 seconds.

MINUTE 3

Under-knee pass

Again, this move is working on your balance and core stability, as you need to be secure on one leg before you can safely pass the cushion beneath. If you are still working on your core stability, you may need to do this exercise close to a wall, so you can touch it with your fingertips if necessary. And, obviously, this move is great for your coordination.

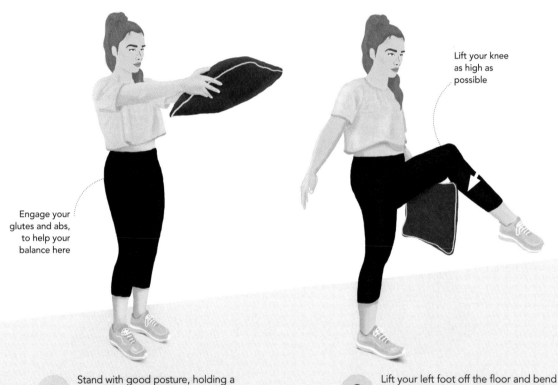

Lift your knee as high as possible

Engage your glutes and abs, to help your balance here

1 Stand with good posture, holding a cushion out straight in front of you. Your arms should be parallel to the floor, so try not to let them drop lower.

2 Lift your left foot off the floor and bend the leg at the knee, getting it as high as possible. With your left arm, take the cushion out to your left side.

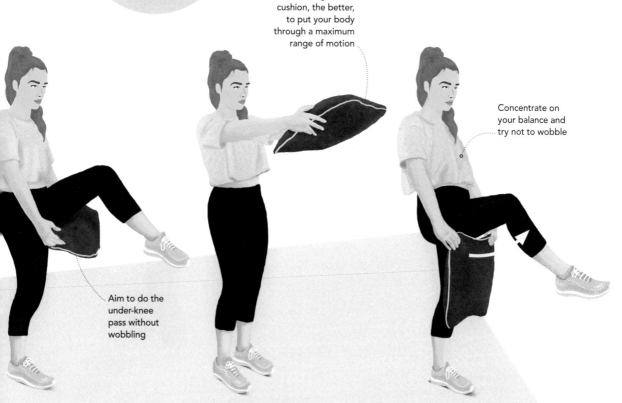

The higher the
cushion, the better,
to put your body
through a maximum
range of motion

Concentrate on
your balance and
try not to wobble

Aim to do the
under-knee
pass without
wobbling

3 Pass the cushion
under your bent leg
and take it with your
right hand.

4 Bring your left foot
back down to the
ground, landing
softly rather than
stamping.

5 Reverse the move, lifting
your right leg and passing
the cushion from right to left.
Repeat, alternating legs, for
60 seconds.

MINUTE 4

Touch down

Practising this touch down is great for your balance, and also works on leg strength and core stability. You will be putting your body through a hefty 90-degrees of Sagittal (backward and forward) motion (see p68), which is difficult to do. Your aim here is to complete the move in a controlled and elegant manner, but don't worry if you're not ballerina-like the first time; as you progress, you'll work up to a smooth movement.

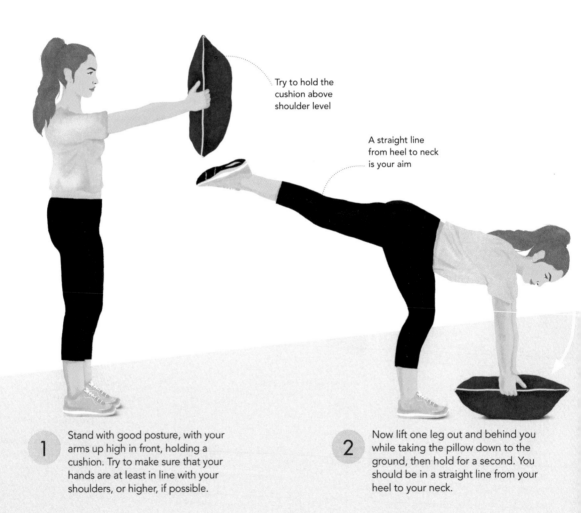

Try to hold the cushion above shoulder level

A straight line from heel to neck is your aim

1. Stand with good posture, with your arms up high in front, holding a cushion. Try to make sure that your hands are at least in line with your shoulders, or higher, if possible.

2. Now lift one leg out and behind you while taking the pillow down to the ground, then hold for a second. You should be in a straight line from your heel to your neck.

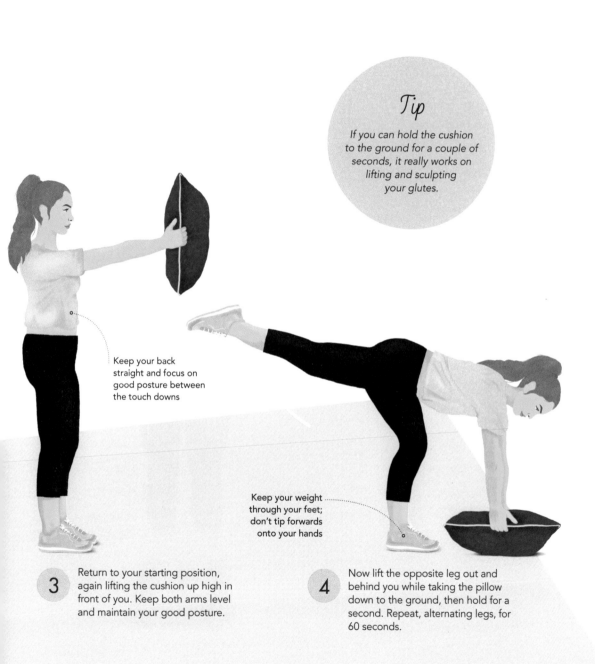

Tip

If you can hold the cushion to the ground for a couple of seconds, it really works on lifting and sculpting your glutes.

Keep your back straight and focus on good posture between the touch downs

Keep your weight through your feet; don't tip forwards onto your hands

3 Return to your starting position, again lifting the cushion up high in front of you. Keep both arms level and maintain your good posture.

4 Now lift the opposite leg out and behind you while taking the pillow down to the ground, then hold for a second. Repeat, alternating legs, for 60 seconds.

MINUTE 5
Stability punch

Try this if you want to improve both your endurance and your balance. It's also incredible for sculpting your waist and arms. Standing on the cushion means your abs and legs get a great workout, as they are forced to act like an anchor, while you are also having to recruit lots of muscles to help stabilize your body as you punch out those arms.

Tip

Focus on keeping your feet, knees, and hips facing forwards, so you are only rotating from your waist up.

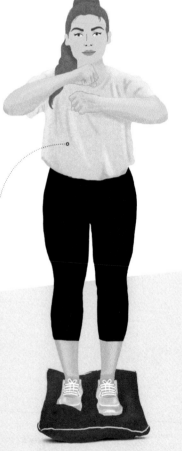

Try not to wobble; focus on keeping your lower body still throughout the move

1 Stand in the middle of a cushion with good posture, keeping a slight bend in your knees. Bring your arms up to your chest, fists clenched and ready to punch!

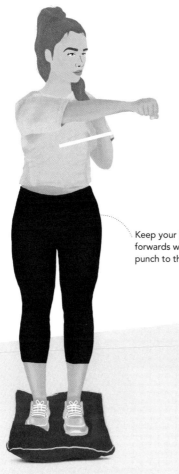

Don't forget your stance while you are punching; keep it stable throughout

Keep your hips facing forwards while you punch to the side

2 Now simply imagine you are boxing and punch each arm back and forth, aiming to go from one side to the other so your right punch goes towards the left and vice versa.

3 Keep your lower body still and stable as you punch from side to side. Repeat, alternating arm punches, for 60 seconds.

MINUTE 6

Lunge & twist

Doing this exercise often will be great for your lower body endurance. The Frontal (lateral) and Transverse (rotational) planes of motion (see p68) are combined in this move, so it's great for the muscles all around your legs. Meanwhile, adding the extended arm twist is superb for your flexibility, and for waist shaping. If you are a runner – or intending to become one – it is so important to build up strength in your lower body, to support tendons and joints as you run.

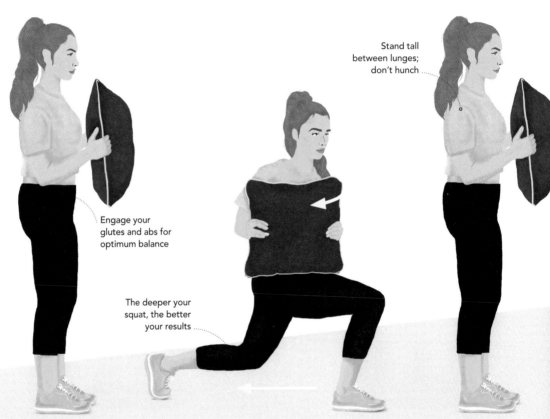

Stand tall between lunges; don't hunch

Engage your glutes and abs for optimum balance

The deeper your squat, the better your results

1 Stand with good posture, holding a cushion in front of you, close to your body.

2 Take a deep step back with your left foot, so you come into a lunge position. Keep the cushion at the same height, but bring it as far as you can around to your right. Hold for a second.

3 Bring the cushion back to the centre, then push off from your right heel and come back to your standing position, still with the cushion held in front.

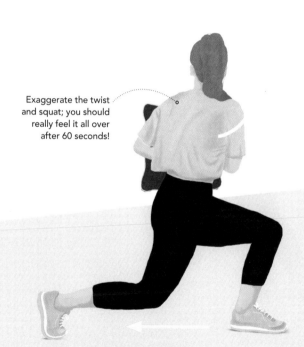

Exaggerate the twist and squat; you should really feel it all over after 60 seconds!

Keep your core muscles engaged and try not to wobble

4 Take a deep step back with your right foot, so you come into a lunge position. Keep the cushion at the same height, but bring it as far as you can around to your left. Hold for a second.

5 Bring the cushion back to the centre, then push off from your left heel and come back to your standing position, still with the cushion held in front. Keep alternating from side to side for 60 seconds.

MINUTE 7
HIIT knee crunch

A power move that is a great stress-buster – really feel it as you "kick" the cushion with your knee. It helps build endurance and strength through your legs, which is useful for joint stability. This exercise also gives your abs an amazing workout at the same time, as you need to engage them to bring your knee up high and hard. Plus, like all the moves in this workout, it does wonders for your balance.

Focus on your intent: you are really going to hit this thing hard

Tip

The faster you do this, the harder it is, so go for gold, especially as it is the last exercise in this routine.

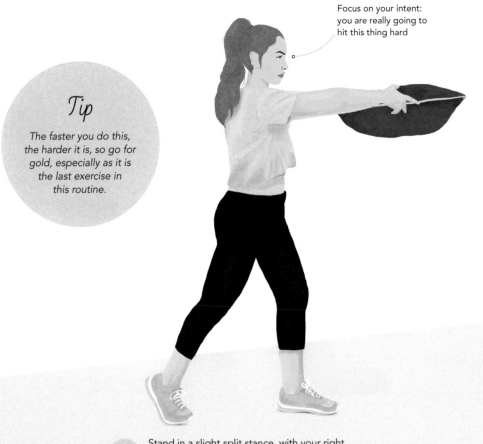

1   Stand in a slight split stance, with your right foot slightly behind you and both feet hip-width apart. Hold a cushion slightly over to your right and just above hip height (if you are very flexible, you can lift it to chest height).

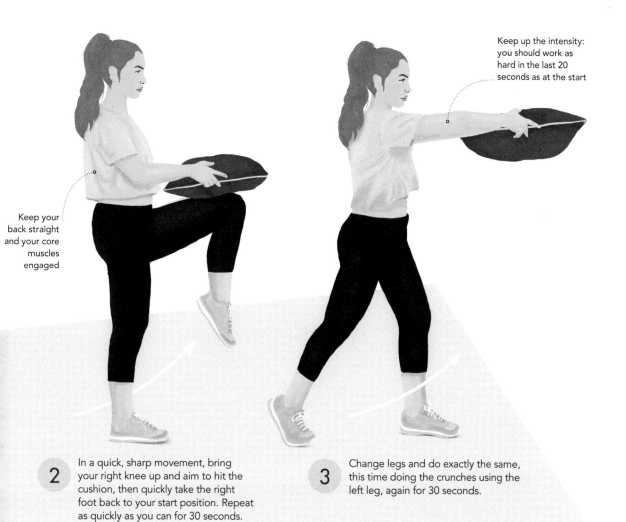

Keep up the intensity: you should work as hard in the last 20 seconds as at the start

Keep your back straight and your core muscles engaged

2 In a quick, sharp movement, bring your right knee up and aim to hit the cushion, then quickly take the right foot back to your start position. Repeat as quickly as you can for 30 seconds.

3 Change legs and do exactly the same, this time doing the crunches using the left leg, again for 30 seconds.

SUPER-CHARGE YOUR
SUPER-HEALTH-FIX WORKOUT

7 TIPS

1 ROLL WITH IT.
Swap a chair that you sit on daily
– even the chair you use at your desk at
work – for a stability ball instead. If you
are sitting on a chair, your body is
static. However, while you are sitting on
a ball, you are helping to improve your
core stability. The reason is that, when
you are on an unstable surface such as
a ball, you have to use extra muscles to
anchor yourself in place. It's the same
reason you work harder in this workout
when you stand on a cushion; you are
having to constantly activate your deep
abdominal muscles to help support
you and hold you in place. Your core
strength is vital, not just for sports, but
for your overall health, and these
muscles are especially important for
maintaining fitness as we age.

2 BE A FLAMINGO.
When you find you are standing for
periods of time, be a secret flamingo
and slightly lift one foot off the ground.
Nobody needs to know! Stand on one
leg, as this will help with your balance.
Do be sure to keep switching legs, to
keep the pressure off one side. A great
time for this is if you are queuing
(waiting in line) at the shops.
Remember to activate your glutes
and abs, to keep you balanced, and
to give them a workout, too.

3 BAN THE BANNISTERS.
Next time you are heading up stairs,
avoid the handrail and concentrate on
walking up just with the power of your
amazing legs. This way you will help to
improve your balance while creating
even more power and endurance
through your entire lower body.

Q&A

*I want to start running
but I find it so hard that I give
up. Where should I start?*

Often, would-be runners try to run too far. So
forget the miles and focus on minutes! Even if
it is 1 minute of running, then 3 of walking,
that is a training session. You'll gradually be
able to run for longer. Plus, this 7-minute
workout is great for increasing
fitness and endurance, so runs
will start feeling easier.

4 BE A "GLASS HALF FULL" PERSON.

Being healthy and fit also means having a positive attitude, so don't forget about the mental side of your health. Luckily, we are all more and more realizing the vital role that this plays in overall wellbeing. We can all help ourselves out by concentrating on being more optimistic. So always try to see your glass as half full. Remember that your mind is constantly feeding your body, so keep telling your mind how powerful and strong your body is.

5 SUPER-CHARGE YOUR NUTRITION.

Aim to be a lots-more-than-5-a-day eater. The common yardstick is to aim for 5 fruits and vegetables a day, though many believe that the true number should be considerably higher than that. If you aim high this way, you know you are eating a rich, nutritionally dense diet, and the healthier your diet is, the more impact it has on your physical performance and ability. Imagine your favourite athlete the day before they are performing in a big event: they will eat super-healthy food because it is quality fuel. So treat yourself and eat like your favourite sports star. And remember to eat the rainbow: the more different colours of vegetables you include in your diet, the better for your health, as the colours come from trace minerals.

Q&A

What is a good post-workout snack?

Natural protein. (So many people think they need protein powders, bars, or supplements.) Natural foods are healthiest and cheapest. Here are some good examples:
*Wholegrain crackers with hummus
A couple of dates, sliced open, pitted, and stuffed with a little nut butter
Small pot of Greek yogurt with berries
Banana and a handful of almonds
Chicken breast in wholemeal pitta*

6 PLAY BALL.

Grab a small bouncy ball, then find a convenient wall and space where you can throw and catch, without annoying the neighbours. This will get your heart rate up and work on your balance and motor skills, as well as all the planes of motion through which your body can work. Aim to do 30 catches every day.

7 COMMIT TO A GOAL.

As you are doing the super-health training this week, why not set yourself a goal, such as a 5K charity race. You'll notice a difference in your fitness from this week, and remember: you can do anything you put your mind to. So be brave and sign up to a new challenge – you will surprise yourself.

THE RECIPES

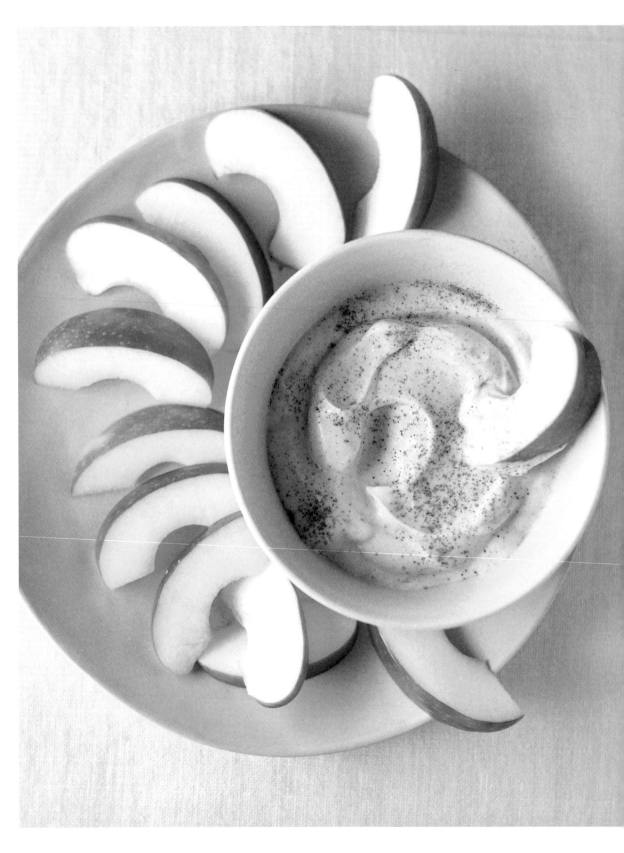

FLUFFY CINNAMON NUT BOWL & APPLE DIPPERS

This super-quick and utterly scrumptious breakfast is ready in a matter of minutes, and with just a few ingredients, it is also budget friendly. It has plenty of protein in both the yogurt and the nut butter, which keep you fuller for longer. The apple dippers ensure you also get a good amount of fibre. If you are vegan, use a dairy-free yogurt instead. Switch up the spices and nut butters for some variety: try almond butter and add a scattering of ground ginger.

INGREDIENTS

150g pot (5½oz/
   generous ½ cup)
   plain Greek yogurt
1 tbsp peanut butter,
   crunchy or smooth,
   as you prefer
1 tsp honey, plus extra
   to taste
pinch of ground
   cinnamon
1 apple

METHOD

1 Put the yogurt, peanut butter, honey, and cinnamon in a bowl. Using a whisk or a fork, whisk together until the mixture becomes slightly fluffy.

2 Wash, core, and slice up the apple, and get ready to start this divine, healthy, protein-packed breakfast. If you want a little more sweetness, just add a bit more honey.

Breakfast

CHERRY-&-BERRY GOLDEN GRANOLA

This big batch of granola will last a couple of weeks if you store it in an airtight container. You could sprinkle it into yogurt, or just add your favourite milk. You could even try (and trust me, this works) pouring a little orange juice over it. Make sure, though, that the juice is not high in sugar. Because the main ingredient is oats – good carbohydrates – this granola will help boost your energy levels. Ready-made granola can often be very high in sugar, so by making it yourself you are in control of exactly what is going in. You have so many incredible benefits from the nutrients here: vitamin C and fibre from the cherries; healthy fats, magnesium and zinc from the pumpkin seeds; while flax is amazing for your heart.

INGREDIENTS

300g (10oz/3 cups) rolled oats

50g (1¾oz/⅓ cup) dried pitted cherries

50g (1¾oz/½ cup) mixed berries

30g (1oz/¼ cup) pumpkin seeds

30g (1oz/scant ¼ cup) sunflower seeds

2 tbsp golden flaxseeds

2 tbsp good-quality flavourless oil

up to 2 tsp honey

METHOD

1 Preheat the oven to 180°C (350°F/Gas 4).

2 Put the oats, cherries, berries, and all 3 types of seeds in a bowl. Pour in the oil, then stir in the honey.

3 Spoon the mixture onto a baking sheet lined with baking parchment, sprinkling it out evenly. Bake for 30–40 minutes, stirring every 10 minutes. If you like it a bit more crispy, cook it a little longer, just be sure to not burn it. Allow to cool and store in an airtight container.

HERBY EGG WRAP WITH LIME AVOCADO WHIP

This is a game-changer. If you want a low-calorie, healthy start that just screams goodness (and can be made in a matter of minutes) then you will love it. It's packed full of high-quality ingredients that are going to keep you feeling fabulous all day long. Avocados are extremely high in antioxidants and especially lutein, which is essential for good eye health.

INGREDIENTS

1 large egg

pinch of mixed herbs
   (optional)

extra seasoning (such as
   chilli flakes/crushed red
   pepper, or paprika)

1 avocado

½–1 lime

METHOD

1 Break the egg into a bowl and beat it lightly with the mixed herbs, and / or seasoning of your choice.

2 Place a non-stick frying pan over a medium heat. Pour in the egg mixture and cook, turning it after a minute to cook the other side. Allow to cool.

3 Peel the avocado, remove the stone, and place the flesh in a blender. Slice the lime in half and squeeze in the juice (for less of a zing just use half the lime). Blend for a couple of minutes, or until smooth and silky. (If you don't have a blender, you can just mash it in a bowl.)

4 Simply spoon the avocado whip evenly down the centre of the egg wrap, then roll it up and enjoy.

Breakfast

OVERNIGHT COFFEE & CRANBERRY OATS

It's so easy to make healthy eating part of your life when you discover these oats. Plus it doubles up as coffee and breakfast in one! Make it before you go to bed, so you are super-prepared the next morning with a delicious breakfast you can grab on the go. To store it overnight, it would be good if you have a Mason jar, or simply a large glass. Oats are an amazing source of carbs and fibre and are also high in protein, so having them for breakfast is a great way to fuel your body for the day ahead.

INGREDIENTS

handful of rolled oats

1 cup of coffee, as you
    prefer to take it

handful of cranberries

pinch of ground
    cinnamon, plus extra
    to serve

2 tsp honey, plus extra
    to serve

1 banana

METHOD

1 Place the oats in a jar or bowl. Then make your cup of coffee as usual. Simply pour it over your oats and mix together, then stir in the cranberries, cinnamon, and honey. Cover and put in the fridge overnight.

2 In the morning, give it a bit of a stir and you are good to go. Slice in the banana and serve with a drizzle of honey and another pinch of cinnamon.

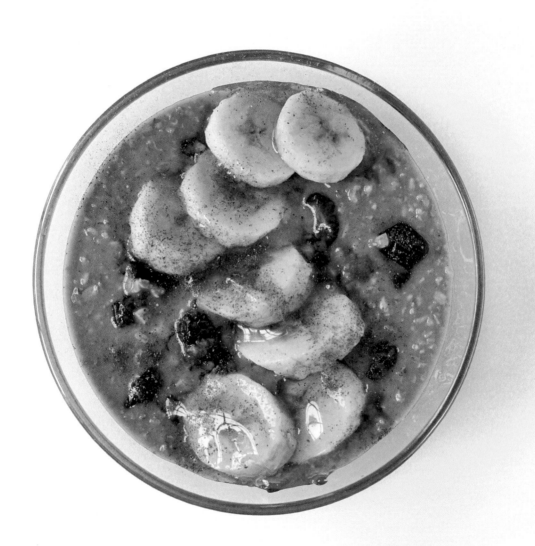

Breakfast

SPINACH & PEPPER QUICHE CUP

Get ready for another super-quick breakfast that you can cook in minutes. It is full of goodness and you can take and eat it anywhere. Eggs are high in protein and very satisfying, plus this is bursting full of protein, minerals, and vitamins. The spinach, especially, is packed with vitamins A and C as well as potassium, which is so good for your blood pressure.

INGREDIENTS

2 handfuls of spinach

1 medium egg

½ red (bell) pepper, deseeded and finely chopped

½ green (bell) pepper, deseeded and finely chopped

seasoning of your choice, such as chilli flakes/ crushed red pepper, dried herbs, or chopped herb leaves

METHOD

1 Wash the spinach well, place it in a microwaveable bowl with a little water, then cover and microwave on High for a couple of minutes. The leaves will wilt. Drain off the water, being very careful of the steam as you can easily burn yourself.

2 Crack the egg into a cup and mix thoroughly, then add both types of pepper and the wilted spinach, plus any seasoning you want. Mix it all together.

3 Microwave on High for about 3 minutes, or until the egg is thoroughly cooked.

4 It will be piping hot, so allow it to cool. Grab a spoon and eat from the cup, or take it with you to eat on the go.

CREAMY MUSHROOMS ON SOURDOUGH

This speedy, easy-to-make savoury breakfast gives you a boost of vitamin D thanks to the mushrooms, a fat-soluble vitamin that's essential to help our bodies absorb calcium and keep our bones strong. Sourdough bread has been fermented, so is both healthy for your gut and easier to digest than other breads. Enjoy this nutrient-rich plateful that will leave you pleasantly full right up until lunch, but not stuffed.

INGREDIENTS

several mushrooms,
   finely sliced
pinch of dried thyme,
   or 1 tsp chopped
   thyme leaves
slice of sourdough bread
1 tbsp reduced-fat cream
   cheese (vegans should
   omit this, or use vegan
   cream cheese)

METHOD

1 Place a non-stick frying pan over a medium heat, add the sliced mushrooms, stirring constantly, then the thyme. Stir until the mushrooms are cooked: they will throw out some moisture, then absorb it again, and take on some golden colour. Remove from the heat.

2 Meanwhile, toast the bread.

3 In a bowl, mix the mushrooms and cream cheese. Now pile this onto your sourdough toast.

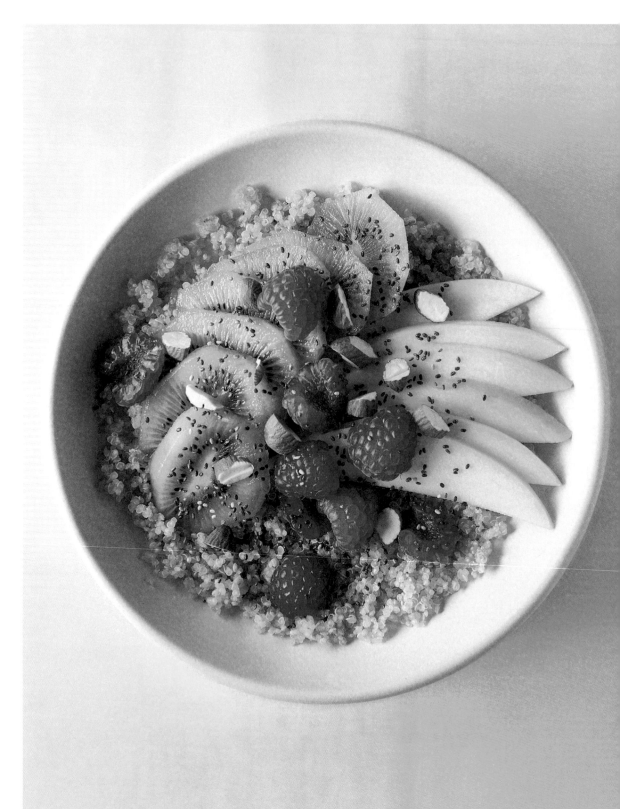

BREAKFAST BUDDHA BOWL

A super-pretty breakfast that tastes as good as it looks. It is bursting with antioxidants and has lots of health benefits, including the fact that it is amazing for helping to promote radiant skin. Normally, Buddha bowls are savoury and eaten for lunch, but they are a fun way to kick-start a healthy day and having them sweet works just as well. Get creative and try other fruits, and perhaps a little nut butter. The main ingredient here is quinoa. This supergrain is a healthy plant protein with a similar texture to couscous and a deliciously nuttier flavour, plus it is simple to prepare. It contains all 9 essential amino acids, making this the perfect protein-power bowl to keep you energized until lunch.

INGREDIENTS

40g (1¼oz/⅓ cup)
   raw quinoa
1 tsp honey
several raspberries
1 kiwi fruit, peeled
   and sliced
several slices of mango
several almonds, with
   skins on
sprinkling of chia seeds

METHOD

1 First, thoroughly rinse the quinoa, then put it into a saucepan and cover with water. Bring to the boil, then reduce the heat, and allow to simmer for 15 minutes, until soft, or the water is fully absorbed. Fluff it up with a fork and mix in the honey.

2 Put the sweetened quinoa into a breakfast bowl.

3 Now you can get decorative with your toppings! Place the fruit on top with the almonds and finish with the chia seeds.

Lunch

HERB-STUFFED COURGETTES

Courgettes (zucchini) are rich in antioxidants, which makes these vegetables a great choice to help look after your skin. This recipe is slightly more complicated than my usual meals, but it shouldn't take you long and the results are well worth the extra effort.

INGREDIENTS

2 large courgettes
 (zucchini)
1 medium egg,
 lightly beaten
50g (1¾oz/½ cup)
 wholemeal (whole-
 wheat) breadcrumbs
1 small garlic clove,
 finely chopped
pinch of dried
 mixed herbs
1 tbsp olive oil
handful of finely grated
 Parmesan cheese

METHOD

1 Preheat the oven to 200°C (400°F/Gas 6). Bring a large saucepan of water to the boil. Carefully lower the whole courgettes into the water, cook for 5 minutes, drain, then leave until cool.

2 Halve the courgettes lengthways and, with a teaspoon, remove the seeds and some of the flesh, to leave hollow shells. Place the seeds and flesh in a bowl, add the egg, breadcrumbs, garlic, and herbs, and mix.

3 Heat the oil in a frying pan and add the breadcrumb mixture. Cook, stirring, until golden, then spoon into the courgette halves, sprinkling the Parmesan on top.

4 Place on a baking tray (baking pan) and bake for 20 minutes, or until golden brown.

MUSHROOM STROGANOFF

Mushrooms are incredibly good for your bone health, as well as for your heart. I've suggested smoked paprika here, though it's helpful to know that you can buy this in hot or sweet varieties, so make sure to read the package before you spend your money, and get your favourite spice.

INGREDIENTS

1 tbsp olive oil

2 spring onions
(scallions),
finely chopped

2 garlic cloves,
finely grated

500g (1lb 2oz/6½ cups)
mushrooms, sliced

2 tsp smoked paprika

freshly ground black
pepper

100g (3½oz/scant ½ cup)
crème fraîche, or
soured cream

handful of coriander
(cilantro) leaves

2 portions cooked brown
rice or whole-wheat
spaghetti, to serve

METHOD

1 Heat the oil in a frying pan and add the spring onions and garlic. Cook until they are soft and transparent.

2 Add the mushrooms gradually and cook down for 5–10 minutes. Add the paprika, pepper, and crème fraîche. Reduce the heat and simmer for 5 minutes.

3 Add the coriander and serve with brown rice or whole-wheat spaghetti.

Tip

You could serve this with Courgette Noodles (see p194) instead of regular spaghetti, for a lighter meal packed with vegetables.

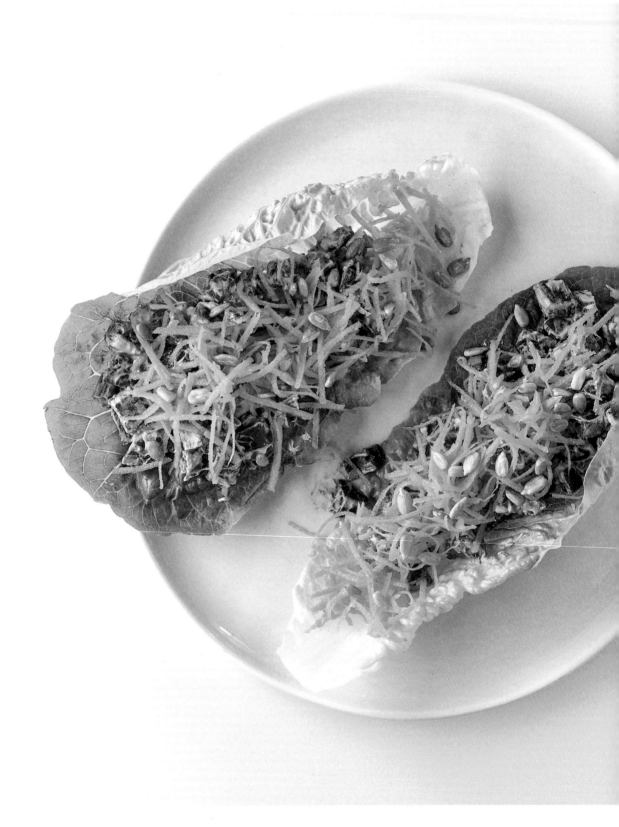

BEETROOT & CARROT WRAPS

Replacing traditional wraps with lettuce leaves means a lot more vitamins and minerals for you, as well as fewer carbs. The same trick works in the evening, too, for burgers or chicken wraps, and especially suits spicy south-east Asian-style skewers, as wrapping food in edible leaves is a traditional way of eating there. These are great to take in a lunch box to work. You can prepare them the night before and store them in the fridge.

INGREDIENTS

2 cooked beetroots (beets), finely chopped or coarsely grated
1 tbsp reduced-fat cream cheese
2 large lettuce leaves
1 carrot, finely grated
pinch of sunflower seeds

METHOD

1 In a bowl, mix the beetroot with the cream cheese, making a creamy pink paste.

2 Lay the large lettuce leaves flat on a work surface.

3 Divide the beetroot mixture in half and spread evenly over both leaves. Sprinkle evenly with the grated carrot and sunflower seeds.

4 Now roll up the lettuce to make rolls, using a cocktail stick to hold them together, if you want.

Lunch

BAKED SWEET POTATO WITH RAINBOW SLAW

Sweet potatoes are sweet in many ways: not only because of how they taste, but also because they are an excellent source of vitamin A, which helps keep your skin glowing and healthy. They are not actually a type of potato, despite the name, but are in fact more closely related to root vegetables such as carrots or parsnips, which is why they have a low glycaemic index rating (so they won't cause a spike in your blood sugar).

INGREDIENTS

1 portion-sized sweet
   potato, scrubbed
¼ red cabbage
1 small carrot
1 apple, cored
2 spring onions
   (scallions),
   finely chopped
150g pot (5½oz/
   generous ½ cup)
   plain low-fat yogurt
pinch of poppy seeds

METHOD

1 Preheat the oven to 180°C (350°F/Gas 4).

2 Bake the sweet potato for 40 minutes, or until tender right through to the centre.

3 Meanwhile, prepare the slaw: grate the red cabbage, carrot, and apple, and mix in a bowl with the spring onions. Stir in the yogurt.

4 Open up the sweet potato, spoon in the rainbow slaw, and sprinkle with poppy seeds.

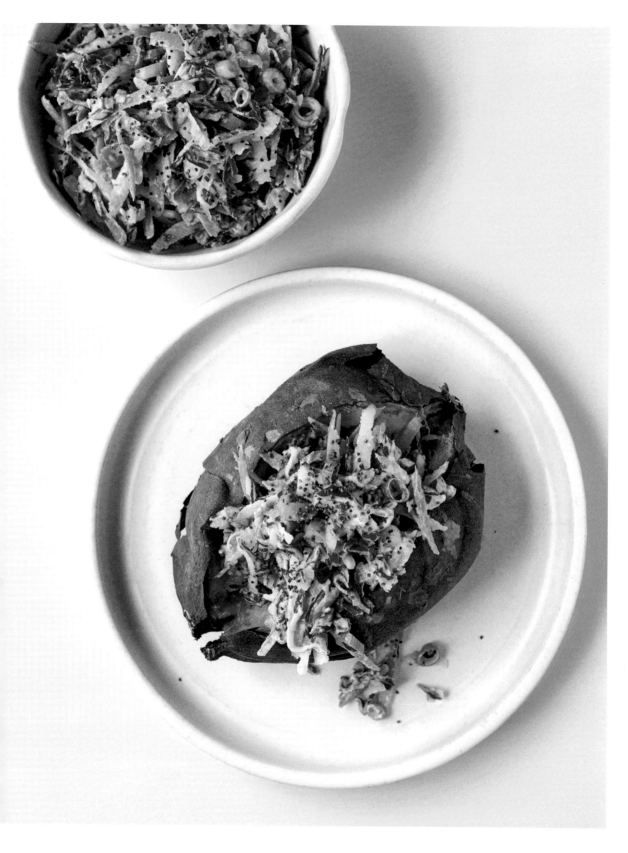

Lunch

MANGO, GUACAMOLE & BLACK BEAN SALAD

This easy-to-make salad is delicious and the beans make it very good for your digestive health, as well as more filling. This is an excellent choice during spring, when mango is in season and especially delectable, while the eye-popping orange, green, and purple-black colours will help cheer up the gloomiest weather.

INGREDIENTS

1 small mango, peeled, stoned, and chopped

½ cucumber, chopped

1 small avocado, peeled, stoned, and chopped

1 small red onion, chopped

½ x 400g can of black beans (1¼ cups), drained and rinsed

juice of 1 lime

1 slice of wholemeal (whole-wheat) sourdough bread

handful of coriander (cilantro) leaves

METHOD

1 Place the mango, cucumber, avocado, onion, and black beans in a bowl, then squeeze over the lime juice.

2 Toast the bread, then crumble it up and sprinkle on top. Scatter with the coriander and serve.

Tip

You can swap black beans for kidney beans (just stick to the same quantity), or even add a sprinkling of prawns (shrimp).

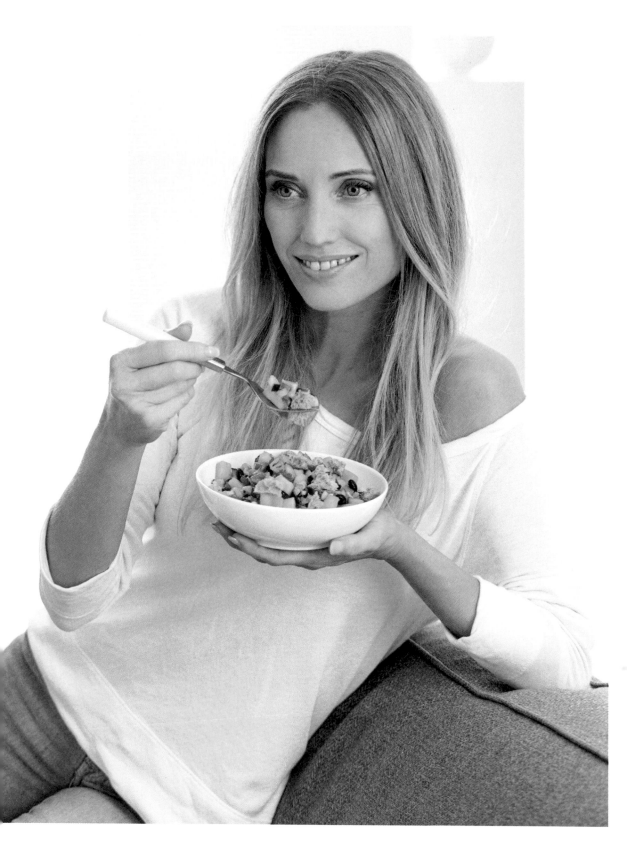

Lunch

WHIPPED FETA TOASTIE WITH BALSAMIC BERRIES

This looks like and tastes like the most indulgent treat, but you can confidently enjoy it knowing it is bursting full with nutritious goodness. The feta and avocado are both full of good fats, which your body needs to function at its peak, while the balsamic glaze adds a welcome touch of sweetness and the strawberries their wonderful sweet acidity.

INGREDIENTS

1 slice of wholemeal
   (whole-wheat)
   sourdough bread,
   or rye bread
handful of feta cheese,
   chopped into cubes
1 small avocado, peeled,
   stoned, and mashed
handful of strawberries,
   sliced
2 tsp balsamic glaze
   (optional)
leaves from 1 mint sprig
pinch of chia seeds, or
   poppy seeds

METHOD

1 Preheat the grill (broiler, or toaster oven) and lightly toast the bread.

2 Put the feta in a blender and blitz (whip) to create a whipped texture.

3 Spread the toast with the mashed avocado, then add the strawberries, then the whipped feta. Drizzle with the balsamic glaze, if you like.

4 Now place under the heat and cook until the feta turns a lovely golden brown. Tear over the mint leaves and sprinkle with the seeds to serve.

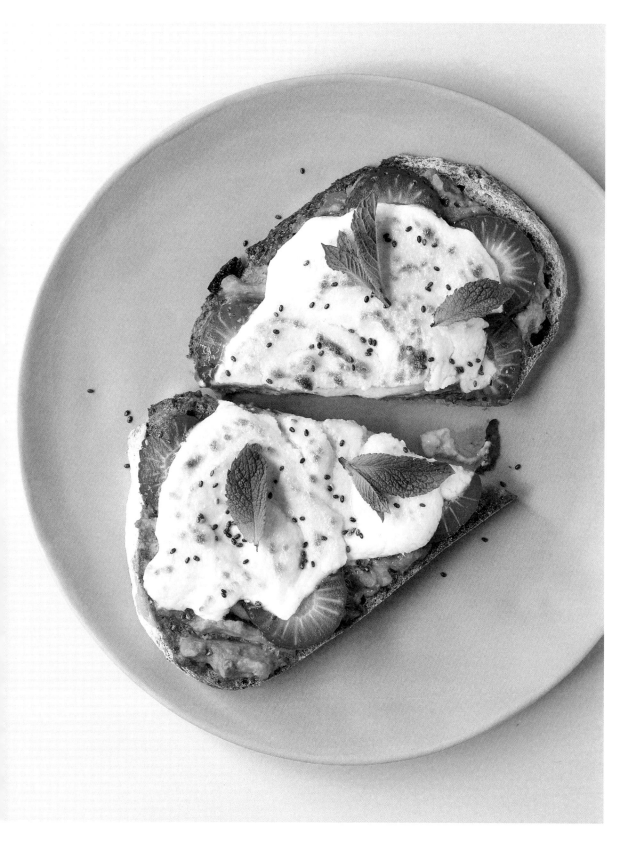

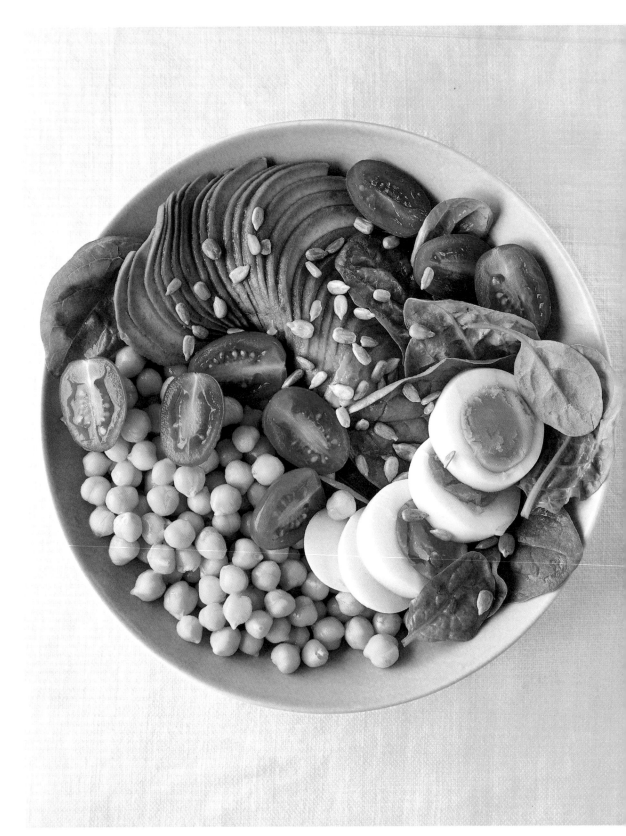

PROTEIN BOWL

This is full of superfoods, along with plenty of protein to keep you energized and feeling satisfied for hours. The good fats from the avocado will help your joints to function at their best. Add a sprinkle of balsamic vinegar, if you would like a bit of dressing.

INGREDIENTS

2 handfuls of
   spinach leaves
handful of cherry
   tomatoes, sliced
½ x 400g can of
   chickpeas (1¼ cups),
   drained and rinsed
1 hard-boiled medium
   egg, sliced
1 small avocado, peeled,
   stoned, and chopped

METHOD

1 Place some of the spinach leaves in a bowl, then a few tomato slices, several chickpeas, a couple of slices of the boiled egg, then the avocado.

2 Keep layering up the ingredients – or just arrange them alongside each other – until you've used them up.

Tip

If you prefer, swap the egg for roughly the same amount of chopped cooked chicken breast.

Snacks

CHOCOLATE BANANA MUG CAKE

This quick, easy cake with just 3 ingredients is a delicious near-enough instant snack. It's high in potassium and great for your digestion. You can play around with the basic recipe, if you like. Try swapping the chocolate powder for a little maple syrup, and even add some metabolism-boosting spices such as cinnamon, nutmeg, or ginger.

INGREDIENTS

1 banana
2 tsp dark drinking chocolate (chocolate milk) powder
1 medium egg, lightly beaten
flavourless vegetable oil spray
handful of raspberries

METHOD

1 Peel the banana and mash it to a paste in a bowl, so it is nice and creamy, then stir in the drinking chocolate powder. Now pour in the egg and mix all 3 ingredients together until smooth.

2 Spray a microwaveable cup with oil, then pour in the cake batter. Microwave for 1 minute on High, then check it: if the mixture is still soft, cook for another 30 seconds.

3 Allow to cool, as it will be piping hot, then eat straight from the cup – or turn it out onto a small plate if you're feeling fancy – and top it off with the raspberries.

KALE & CHILLI CRISPS

Kale is king, as it is low in calories, yet high in vitamins A, C, and K. These crisps (chips) are super-easy, but you need to watch therm carefully so they don't scorch. Make sure they are cooked in a single layer, as that way they will crisp up both more rapidly and more evenly.

INGREDIENTS

250g bag of curly kale
  (4 cups)
drizzle of olive oil
2 tsp chilli flakes/crushed
  red pepper

METHOD

1 Preheat the oven to 180°C (350°F/Gas 4).

2 Wash the kale and dry it thoroughly. Place it in a large bowl, tearing any big leaves into smaller pieces.

3 Drizzle the oil over, then massage it into the kale. Sprinkle in the chilli flakes and mix well, then spread out in a single layer over a couple of baking trays (baking sheets).

4 Bake for 20 minutes, or until crisp but still green, removing the leaves that turn crisp first from the trays, then leave them all to cool for a few minutes.

Tip

If you want to have a dip with these, then they are very good with mint dressing (see p196).

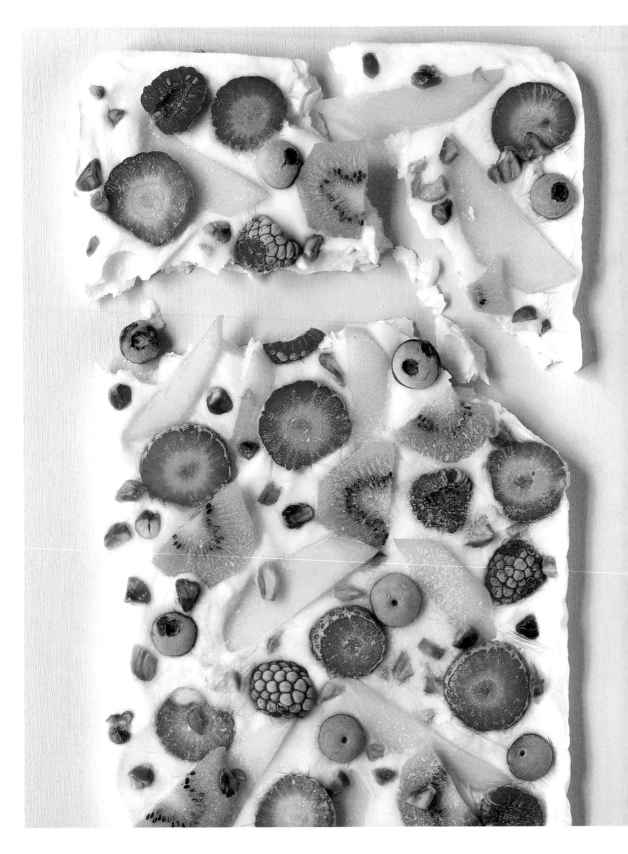

FROZEN BERRY BARK

This sweet treat is a great way of getting in plenty of fruit, while by eating a lot of colours you can be sure of a good mix of vitamins and minerals. If you want to be creative, blitz (purée) red berries such as raspberries in a blender and mix them with the yogurt, to colour it a vibrant pink, or even stir in ½ tsp of cocoa powder instead, before adding the whole fruits.

INGREDIENTS

150g pot (5½oz/
   generous ½ cup)
   plain yogurt
handful of blueberries
1 kiwifruit, peeled
   and sliced
handful of raspberries
small handful of pistachio
   nuts, chopped
handful of sliced mango
handful of sliced
   strawberries

METHOD

1 Line a freezer-proof baking tray (baking sheet) with a sheet of baking parchment.

2 Now pour on the yogurt, spreading it out in a 5mm (¼in) layer. Evenly sprinkle over all the other ingredients, getting a good mix.

3 Place in the freezer and allow to freeze for 3–4 hours.

4 When you want a healthy snack, just head to your freezer and break off some of the berry bark.

Tip

Offer this as a stunning dessert when friends are over. Serve as shards in bowls of plain yogurt. Drizzle with a sauce made of blitzed (puréed) berries and scatter with chopped pistachios. It will look so impressive!

Snacks

RASPBERRY COCONUT ICE CREAM CUPCAKES

These healthy cupcakes contain dates, an excellent substitute for refined sugar and full of nutrients, antioxidants, and fibre. It's always a good idea to use fruit in season – it's both cheaper and tastier – so swap in other ripe fruits when it's not raspberry season.

INGREDIENTS

100g (3½oz/generous ½ cup) pitted dates
80g (2¾oz/¾ cup) walnuts
80g (2¾oz/¾ cup) pecans
60g (2oz/scant ¼ cup) plain Greek yogurt
100g (3½oz/¾ cup) raspberries
1 tsp honey
2 tbsp desiccated coconut (coconut flakes)

METHOD

1 Put the dates into a blender and add the walnuts and pecans. Splash in a little water, then blend to make a nice thick mixture.

2 Remove and spread equally between 8 cupcake cases (baking cups), keeping the mixture about 1cm (½in) deep. Place in the fridge to chill for 7–8 minutes.

3 Now put the yogurt into the blender with the raspberries, honey, and half the coconut. Blend to make a nice creamy mixture.

4 Spread the raspberry mixture evenly over the date bases, using a flat spatula to make the top nice and smooth. Top with the remaining coconut.

5 Now freeze for 4–6 hours.

6 Before serving, remove from the freezer and allow a good 10 minutes to thaw slightly before digging in.

HOT PEA & FETA MELT POT

This super-simple green-and-white pot is very satisfying and delivers plenty of protein, making it a perfect filling healthy snack. If you're vegan, leave out the feta and use a vegan cheese substitute, or replace it with the same amount of smoked tofu, which you can buy from health food shops.

INGREDIENTS

2 tbsp frozen peas
2 small bite-sized cubes
    of feta cheese (or see
    recipe introduction)
several mint leaves,
    finely chopped

METHOD

1 Tip the frozen peas into a saucepan of boiling water and cook for 3 minutes, then drain.

2 Put the peas into a Mason jar or a bowl, then crumble over the feta while the peas are piping hot, so it starts to melt very slightly and become creamy. Sprinkle on the mint leaves.

Tip

You could also make this with edamame beans instead of peas, to give even more vitamins and protein.

BEAN, CUMIN & CHILLI DIP WITH RED CRUDITÉS

Butter beans are an amazing source of protein, fibre, iron, and vitamin B. This recipe makes a nice healthy alternative to regular hummus. We all know we need to eat lots of vegetables, but bear in mind that their colour is also important: the more colours you can eat, the more nutrients you get. I've chosen a pop of red here, but mix it up if this is a frequent snack.

INGREDIENTS

½ x 400g can of white
   butter beans (1¼ cups),
   drained and rinsed
pinch of chilli (chili)
   powder
pinch of ground cumin
sea salt and freshly
   ground black pepper
   (optional)
1 red (bell) pepper, sliced
handful of radishes,
   halved

METHOD

1 Pour the butter beans into a blender and add the spices, with seasoning if you wish. Blend to a paste.

2 Spoon into a bowl and serve up with the red crudités.

Tip

This also makes a great filling to have in a baked sweet potato (see p174).

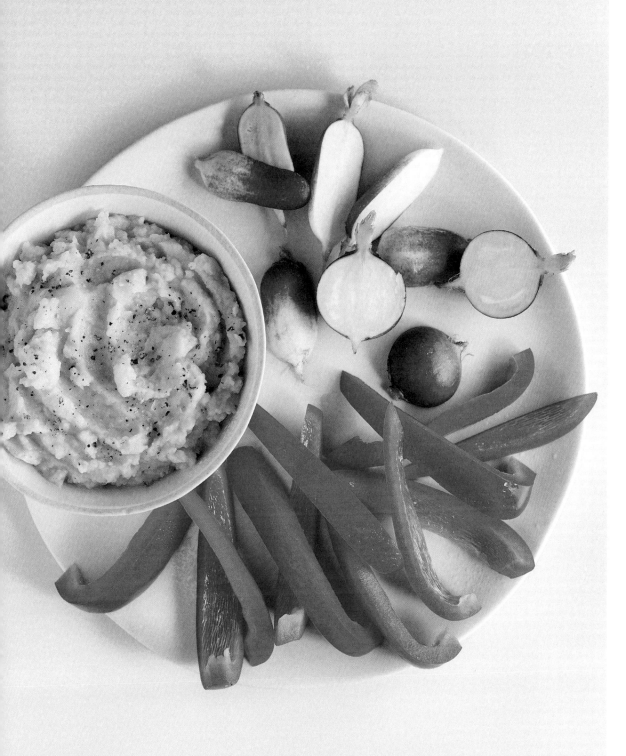

Snacks

RICE PAPER VEGETABLE SPRING ROLLS

A very easy way to make sure you are getting plenty of vegetables. These are an easy snack to prepare ahead and have handy in the office, to stop you reaching for the sugary snacks. Use any combination of vegetables you want, just make sure they have a good crunch, for the best results.

INGREDIENTS

2 sheets of rice paper

1 carrot, cut into matchsticks

¼ cucumber, cut into matchsticks

1 red (bell) pepper, cut into matchsticks

¼ head of lettuce, shredded

2 spring onions (scallions), cut into batons

soy sauce, to serve (optional)

METHOD

1 Fill a small bowl with warm water. Dip in a rice paper sheet for a good minute, until fully moistened, then remove and lay flat on a plate. Do the same with the other rice paper sheet, laying it on a separate plate.

2 Evenly divide the remaining ingredients between both rice paper sheets, laying them in a line down the centres of each sheet. Fold both ends over the filling, to stop it from falling out, then gently roll up, to make spring rolls.

3 Eat with a small dipping bowl of soy sauce, to give an extra wow factor.

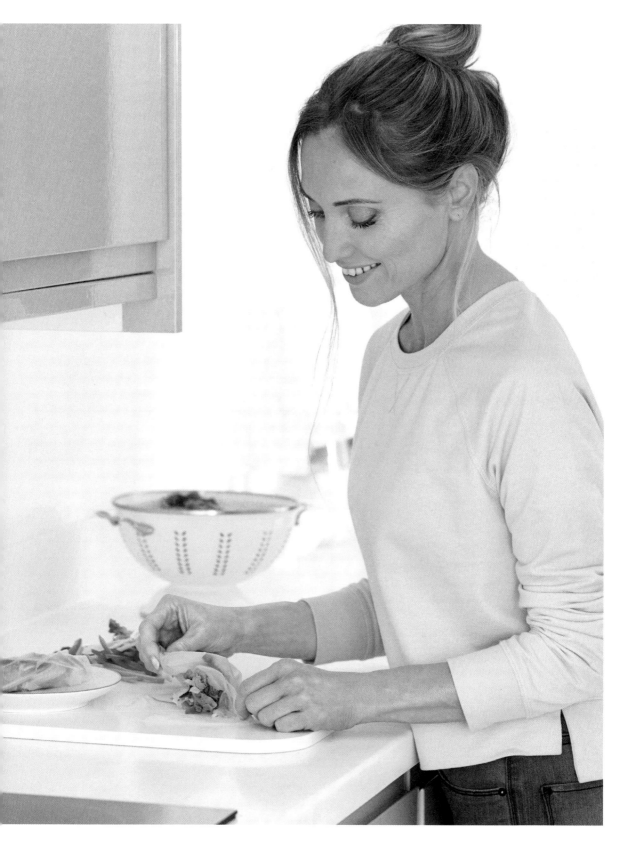

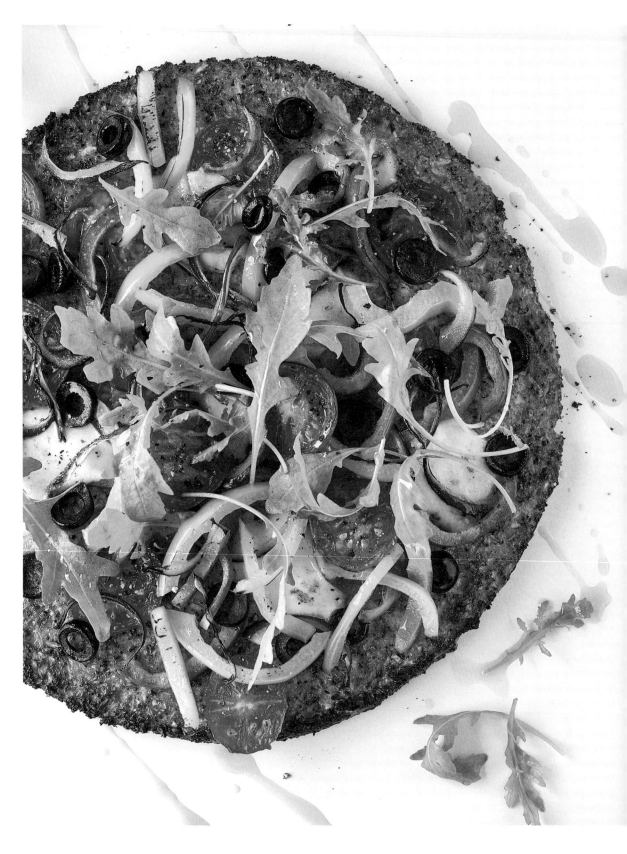

HEALTH-BOOST PIZZA

Trust me: this is so good. You don't even need to be a broccoli lover to enjoy it, as the base tastes divine. It is low-carb, gluten-free, and flourless, so this is a super-healthy pizza that is stuffed full with goodness.

INGREDIENTS

For the base

1 large head of broccoli

2 large eggs

30g (1oz/generous
  ¼ cup) finely grated
  Parmesan cheese

25g (scant 1oz/¼ cup)
  grated mozzarella

1 tsp dried mixed herbs

For the topping

25g (scant 1oz/¼ cup)
  fresh mozzarella, torn

2–3 tomatoes, sliced

1 yellow (bell) pepper

1 green (bell) pepper

1 small red onion, sliced

handful of black olives

a few rocket (arugula)
  leaves and a drizzle of
  extra virgin olive oil, to
  serve (optional)

METHOD

1 Preheat the oven to 200°C (400°F/Gas 6).

2 Trim off the excess broccoli stem and break the head into florets. Peel and finely chop the remaining stem. Place in a food processor and blend until it looks like crumbs. Place into a microwaveable bowl, cover and cook in the microwave on High for about 1½ minutes.

3 In a mixing bowl, beat the eggs, Parmesan, mozzarella, and dried mixed herbs, then stir in the broccoli to form a paste. Season, if you like.

4 Spread out on a sheet of baking parchment to form a 20–25cm (8–10in) pizza base; make sure it is not too thin, or it might burn. Cook in the oven for 10–12 minutes.

5 Remove from the oven and add the torn mozzarella, piling it all over the base, then top with the tomatoes, sliced peppers, red onion, and olives. Bake for 7–10 minutes, or until the mozzarella is golden.

6 It's completely delicious just like this, but you could add a few rocket leaves and drizzle with a good-quality olive oil, if you like.

Dinner

COURGETTE NOODLES & CORIANDER PESTO

This super-quick dish tastes as vibrant as it looks and is full of colourful ingredients, which means it is bursting with antioxidants. Courgettes are super-low-calorie and high in fibre, too. The pop of pink radishes and peppercorns is beautiful against the jade green noodles.

INGREDIENTS

2 courgettes (zucchini), trimmed

2 tbsp good-quality extra virgin olive oil

2 garlic cloves, finely chopped

sea salt and freshly ground black pepper

35g (1¼oz/⅓ cup) pine nuts

2 handfuls of coriander (cilantro)

20g (¾oz/scant ¼ cup) finely grated Parmesan cheese

handful of radishes, finely sliced

1 tsp pink peppercorns

handful of pomegranate seeds

METHOD

1 Preheat the oven to 200°C (400°F/Gas 6).

2 If you have a spiralizer, this is the time to use it to make the courgettes into noodles. If you don't, simply coarsely grate the courgettes.

Transfer the noodles to a baking sheet. Drizzle with half the oil and sprinkle with half the garlic, salt, and pepper. Toss with your hands and spread into an even layer. Roast for 12–15 minutes, until just softened.

3 Meanwhile, heat a small frying pan over a low heat, add the pine nuts and toast until golden, shaking. Put into a food processor with the coriander, Parmesan, the remaining oil and garlic, and blend to a smooth paste.

4 Arrange the noodles in a bowl and top with the pesto, radishes, peppercorns, and pomegranate.

CHEESE & SPINACH BAKE WITH PINE NUTS

A true comfort food dish, with the advantage of being astonishingly healthy. This meal is loaded with spinach, which is packed with potassium, folate, and vitamin C. Add sliced tomatoes to the layers, if you like, for a little extra juiciness.

INGREDIENTS

100g bag of spinach
  leaves (3 cups)
pinch of freshly grated
  nutmeg
1 garlic clove,
  finely chopped
250g (9oz/1 cup)
  cottage cheese
2 medium eggs
sea salt and freshly
  ground black pepper
  (optional)
handful of pine nuts

METHOD

1 Preheat the oven to 180°C (350°F/Gas 4).

2 Put the spinach into a saucepan, cover, and place over a medium heat for about 5 minutes, stirring from time to time, until wilted. Spoon into a sieve and leave to drain until cool enough to handle, then squeeze it in your fists to remove all the excess liquid.

3 In a large bowl, stir the nutmeg and garlic into the cottage cheese.

4 In a separate bowl, beat the eggs and season with salt and pepper, if you wish.

5 Now take a small ovenproof dish. Lay in some spinach, then add a spoonful of the egg, then a layer of the cheese. Keep layering until all the ingredients are used, finishing with a layer of cheese.

6 Scatter with the pine nuts and cook for 20 minutes, or until golden.

Dinner

HALLOUMI KEBABS WITH MINT DRESSING

This easy meal is a great way to get lots of vegetables into a single dish. And remember: the more colours you eat, the more vitamins and minerals you are treating yourself to. Swap the halloumi for chicken, if you prefer.

INGREDIENTS

1 courgette (zucchini)

1 small red onion

1 small green (bell) pepper

60g (2oz/½ cup) halloumi cheese

4 cherry tomatoes

handful of button mushrooms, trimmed

1 wholemeal pitta (whole-wheat pita)

For the mint dressing

1 tbsp plain low-fat yogurt

small handful of finely sliced cucumber

small handful of mint leaves, chopped

sprinkle of chilli (chili) powder (optional)

METHOD

1 Preheat the grill (broiler or toaster oven) to medium. If you have no medium setting, adjust the shelves so the kebabs won't cook too fast. Cut the courgette, onion, pepper, and halloumi into bite-sized chunks.

2 Thread all the vegetables, including the tomatoes and mushrooms, and the halloumi onto a couple of metal skewers. Cook under the grill (broil) for about 8 minutes, turning regularly. Place the pitta under the grill (broiler) for the last couple of minutes, to warm up.

3 Meanwhile, to make the mint dressing, simply stir all the ingredients in a small bowl. Sprinkle with the chilli powder if you want a little extra kick.

4 Serve the skewers drizzled with the dressing, or serve the dressing on the side, if you prefer.

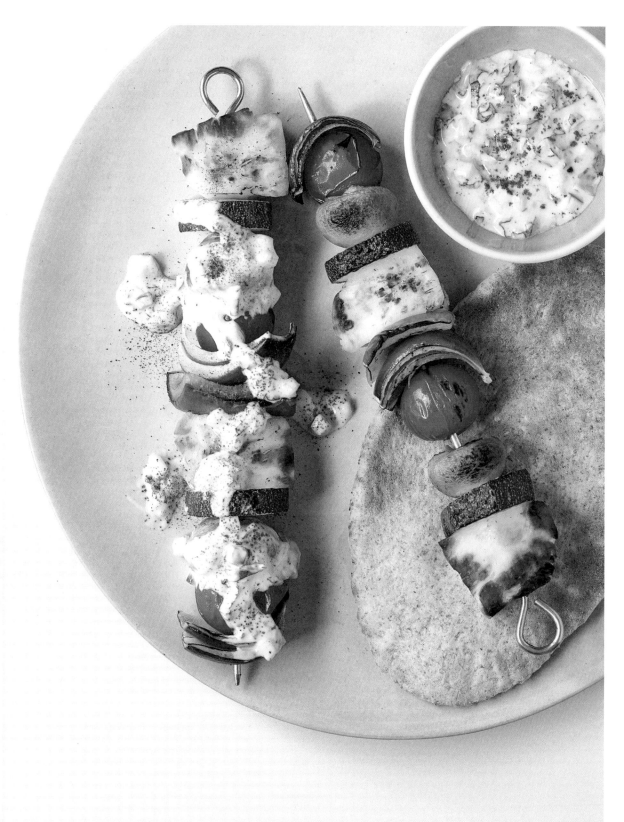

Dinner

SWEET POTATO & PEA CURRY

This is bursting with goodness, as sweet potato is a rich source of vitamin C, which helps boost your immune system and gives your skin a radiant glow.

INGREDIENTS

For the curry

1 tsp good-quality
   vegetable oil
2 tsp mild curry powder
1 small onion,
   finely chopped
300ml (½ pint/1¼ cups)
   vegetable stock
2 large sweet potatoes,
   chopped
200g (7oz) frozen peas
120ml (4fl oz/½ cup)
   canned coconut milk
handful of coriander
   (cilantro) leaves

**For the cauliflower
   "rice"**

½ cauliflower, in florets
2 tbsp finely chopped
   parsley leaves

METHOD

1 Put the oil into a saucepan and stir in the curry powder and onion. Cover and cook for 5 minutes, stirring occasionally, until softened.

2 Now pour in the stock and add the sweet potatoes. Cook until they are tender. Add the peas and cook for another 5 minutes. Pour in the coconut milk and briefly bring to the boil, then scatter with the coriander.

3 Meanwhile, make the cauliflower "rice". Place the cauliflower florets in a blender and blitz (blend) them until they look like rice. Just before the curry is ready, place the "rice" in a microwaveable bowl, cover, and microwave on High for 30–40 seconds. Remove and mix in the parsley, then serve with the curry.

MEDITERRANEAN OMELETTE

Omelettes are a good healthy dinner or lunch choice as they are high in protein and, with this one, I have added some Mediterranean goodness to give it an extra health boost. You can go to town adding spices to this; try chilli flakes (crushed red pepper) or cayenne pepper, for a warming kick.

INGREDIENTS

1 medium egg

1 tsp paprika

small knob (1 tsp) of
   unsalted butter, or
   1 tsp low-calorie oil

small handful of olives

small handful of
   bite-sized cubes
   of feta cheese

small handful of
   semi-dried tomatoes

handful of spinach leaves

METHOD

1 Break the egg into a bowl and whisk in the paprika.

2 Heat the butter or oil in a pan over a medium heat, then pour in the egg and cook.

3 Once half-cooked, scatter over the olives, feta, tomatoes, and spinach, then fold a side over to cover the filling and cook for a minute. Flip over and cook until golden on the other side, then serve.

Tip

Just whisk all the ingredients together and cook it as a Spinach & Pepper Quiche Cup (p166), if you prefer.

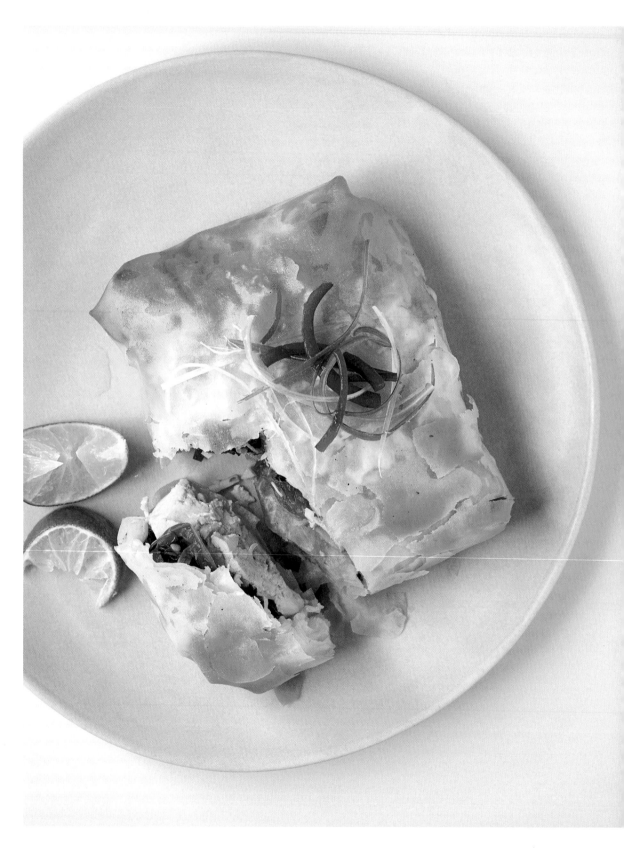

Dinner

ASIAN TOFU TART

Simply divine. The flavours are incredible and the tart contains lots of metabolism-boosting ingredients such as ginger and chilli. Double win! Try marinating the tofu overnight, if you have time, for a fuller flavour.

INGREDIENTS

80g (2¾oz/⅓ cup) firm tofu, drained of liquid

2 tsp soy sauce

2 sheets of filo (phyllo) pastry

1 small red chilli (chile), finely chopped, plus extra to serve

1 spring onion (scallion), finely chopped, plus extra to serve

2.5cm (1in) fresh root ginger, grated

½ garlic clove, finely chopped or grated

handful of coriander (cilantro) leaves, torn

handful of cherry tomatoes, halved

drizzle of good-quality vegetable oil

sea salt and freshly ground black pepper

1 lime, to serve

METHOD

1 Preheat the oven to 200°C (400°F/Gas 6).

2 Put the tofu into a bowl, pour over the soy sauce and allow to marinate. (Do this at least an hour before you plan to cook this meal, if you can.)

3 Line a baking tray with a sheet of baking parchment. Place the 2 sheets of filo pastry on the tray, to form a double layer.

4 Lay the soy-soaked tofu in the centre, then scatter with the chilli, spring onion, ginger, garlic, coriander, and tomatoes. Drizzle with oil and add a little seasoning.

5 Now fold in the ends and make a filo parcel, in much the same way as you'd wrap a birthday present.

6 Cook for about 15 minutes, or until the filo is golden. Squeeze over some lime juice to give it that final zing, and scatter with red chilli and spring onion.

7 healthy

SMOOTHIES

Smoothies are the quickest way to get a whole bunch of nutrients in you. They are a great way to boost health and energy levels, and are amazing for your skin, hair, and nails: one of the best beauty products is our food, as it works from the inside out. For all these recipes, prepare the fruit and veg as necessary, then blend until smooth.

1 GREEN GODDESS

The emerald-green colour shows this is bursting with goodness; specifically vitamins E, C, and K, and folate.

INGREDIENTS

1 small avocado, peeled
   and stoned
1 small apple
¼ cucumber
1 celery stick
handful of seedless grapes
100ml (3½fl oz/scant ½ cup) water
½ lime

2 GORGEOUS GLOW

A vibrant orange smoothie jam-packed with vitamin C, and an extra boost of copper from the ginger.

INGREDIENTS

Serves 1
1 orange
2 carrots
thumbnail-sized piece of fresh
   root ginger, peeled

3 PRETTY IN PINK

This looks super-cute but is also super-hydrating.

INGREDIENTS

handful of strawberries, hulled
½ small watermelon, skin and
   seeds removed
½ lime

5 HEALTH IN A GLASS

Pineapple is high in vitamin C and can help boost your immune system.

INGREDIENTS

¼ pineapple, peeled and cored
3 celery sticks
2 handfuls of spinach leaves
240ml (1 cup) unsweetened
   apple juice

7 LOVE HEART SMOOTHIE

The beetroot contains nutrients that help to keep your blood and heart healthy.

INGREDIENTS

2 small cooked beetroots
   (beets)
1 apple
1 carrot
thumbnail-sized piece of
   fresh root ginger, peeled

4 VERY CHERRY

Cherries contain anthocyanins, powerful antioxidants with anti-inflammatory properties, so can help stiff muscles after working out.

INGREDIENTS

120g (½ cup) pitted cherries
1 small banana

6 BERRY BEAUTY BLAST

Blueberries are packed with antioxidants, which are great to keep us looking radiant.

INGREDIENTS

1 kiwi, peeled
1 pear
handful of blueberries

THE 7-MINUTE BODY PLAN FOR LIFE

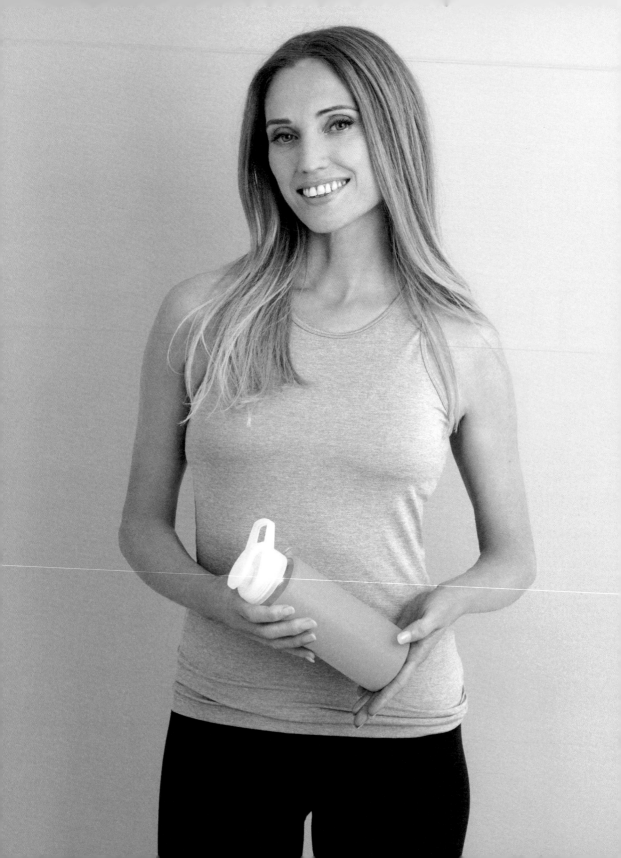

LIFELONG FITNESS
MAINTENANCE

If you've completed the 7 workouts in this book, and followed the extra tips I've given you throughout, I know you'll be feeling amazing. But my job isn't over yet. I've got to make sure you carry on being the best version of you forever.

The most important thing – and I know I've said this before in the book, but it's worth repeating – is to always work out at a time that best suits you. If you are an early-morning person, do the exercises first thing; but if you struggle to get up, work out at lunchtime or in the evening. I can't stress this enough: consistency is key. So establish what time works for you and lock the workouts into your routine.

Keep uppermost in your mind that maintaining a healthy body is a gift from you to you. It's investing in your future health. Having that as a mindset to back up your workouts and healthy eating is a really good motivator. I get emails every day from people who feel the workouts have had a positive impact on their mental and physical health – they've achieved that through healthy eating and exercise.

Get really excited: you've found this 7-minute workout and it's going to work forever. Be really proud that you're feeling great now after just 7 weeks. And know that you want to stay on that road. Believe me, it's far easier to stick on it than

to get off. When you get off track, you tend to eat unhealthily and don't want to exercise, so are less motivated and have less energy. It's a vicious circle, so it's really important to try and stay on track.

Remember: you might have done the Dream arms workout (see p50) and be delighted with the results, but it's important not to do it once and then just stop. To maintain those results, you need to continue the exercises and to keep your whole body healthy, fit, and strong.

A good motivational tip is to reward yourself by season. Each time you finish a workout, add a few coins to a money jar. At the end of each season, use the cash to invest in a nice new bit of fitness gear, to reward yourself for doing well and keep you motivated. Summer coming up? Get a nice vest top. In the winter, get a good pair of longer leggings. It's like going back to school used to be: each season, get a piece of clothing to incentivize you, just as you used to update your pencil case! Remember: you're investing in your future health.

FALLING OFF THE WAGON.

Having said all that, it's vital not to panic if you do come off track every now and then. It's quite normal. The best thing to do is to turn it around: once we feel good, we're more likely to stick to a healthy regime. So set aside one evening to have a bubble bath, paint your nails, or whatever you love best about self care. When you wake up, you'll look better, and will be more likely to get back on the road to health. If you wake up feeling awful, you're far less likely to get that motivation. Don't let the residual negativity of that blow-out, or that week off working out, stop you from getting straight back into shape. If you think you'll never get back to it, that becomes a self-fulfilling prophecy. So think positive, take control, and get back on track.

Why 7 minutes?

As a trainer with many years of experience, I know the most common problem people have with making fitness a habit is time. I tested lots of different workouts online, from 4 minutes to 10 minutes, and the hands-down favourite was 7 minutes. It's enough time to work up a sweat, yet it doesn't sound long or intimidating. It's a sweet spot, the magic 7; a do-able amount of time.

TRAVEL FITNESS.

If you're on holiday or vacation, you can do 7-minute workouts wherever you are. However, you could also swap out the workouts for a week in favour of keeping your step count up. Do plenty of walking, explore your holiday or vacation destination, and let yourself know that as soon as you return home you're getting back into your 7-minute workout routine. Keep control. Know you are going to have those rest times, just keep active, and get back into your schedule once you're back to normality.

CATCH THOSE ZZZS.

Sleep is really important, it's when your body repairs itself. An hour before bedtime, avoid electronic devices and step away from social media. When you're asleep, your body balances out your hormones. If you're sleep-deprived, hunger hormones get confused with tiredness hormones, as your body just tries to give you energy, which leads to overeating. Aim for 7–8 hours of quality sleep each night. You'll find that one of the benefits of exercising is that it will help with sleep, as will healthy eating. And, of course, we all know the power of a relaxing bath, or drops of lavender essential oil on a pillow.

FITNESS AND AGE.

Never think you're getting too old to work out. Exercise is the best medicine for any age. In my workouts, we're using only body weight, so putting no extra pressure through the joints. Whatever age you are, exercise is how to keep your body young. In fact, the older you are, the more you *should* be exercising. Age is simply a number; it's exercise that lowers the risk of getting stressed, having injuries, or becoming ill. If you're 80 and you pick up this book, don't think it's not for you. In fact, you *should* be doing it; exercise will be fantastic for you.

FUEL YOUR WORKOUTS.
As for healthy food, keep it fresh, along with the new workouts you'll be creating (see p210–217). Now you're eating healthily, keep learning: look up new recipes online, every season find new dishes to make, and learn about seasonality in food, because healthy eating and exercise go hand in hand. And encourage your colleagues and friends to do it as well. Go on a long walk together and take turns to make a healthy lunch for the group. Keep eating well, and never try to lose weight if you don't need to.

Long term, keeping your body healthy is about balance. Just remember that treat food is not always unhealthy food – just see my Chocolate Banana Mug Cake or my Raspberry Coconut Ice Cream Cupcakes for proof of that (see p182 and p186). I love pizza, but I will bake a healthy one rather than get a takeaway (see p193). I also love chocolate, and don't beat myself up if I have a bar. It's all about being in control of your lifestyle and, every single day, investing in your health.

A LIFE-LONG PLAN FOR YOUR BODY.
Get really excited that you will be living your healthiest and best life from here on. It is easier

As I know I am going to get fitter, could I increase the amount of training I do in a day?

Yes, if you want to. You could do 2 back-to-back workouts in the morning, or do a second at lunchtime or during the early evening. But only if you want to. These workouts have been designed so just 7 minutes a day will get great results. These exercises still always feel challenging, even as you get fitter, simply because you are using so many muscle groups. So, if you have the urge and lots of energy, then keep going. If not, don't. Listen to your body and do what feels right for it.

than you have ever realized. You don't need the gym. You don't need to spend hours exercising. You don't need to be a master chef. You don't need to spend a fortune on food. Consistency is key. And knowledge is power. You know how to continue, it's all in this book. Once you feel healthy and fit, you will never want to go back to feeling the opposite.

CREATE YOUR OWN
7-MINUTE WORKOUTS

Within this book you have 7 different 7-minute workout routines, which are each meant to be performed for 7 days running. That gives you 7 weeks' worth of training, and you could, of course, choose to then simply keep rotating the workouts. It's the easiest way.

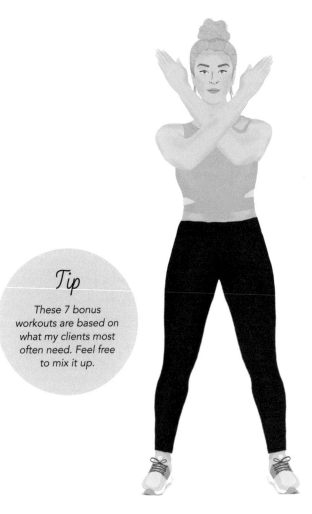

Tip

These 7 bonus workouts are based on what my clients most often need. Feel free to mix it up.

However, you have within this book a total of 49 exercises. Do you know how many different workouts you could do with these? Are you ready for this, because it will blow your mind... I'm not great at numbers, but my nephew is a genius, so I phoned him up and asked how many different sequences you can make. He paused for a second, then said, "It's a very, very big number, let me get back to you." In a matter of minutes he phoned me back with the answer: more than 87 million. Yes I know that is crazy, but it's true. (Don't ask me how he worked it out; my skill set is getting you looking and feeling your best, not maths!)

So you can literally keep creating new 7-minute workouts forever! You will never get bored. To start you off, here are 7 more workouts I've designed especially for you and your lifestyle.

WORKOUT 1: *If you sit down all day*

A 7-minute workout that is all about stretching your muscles, re-aligning your body, and re-energizing you.

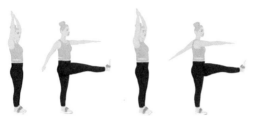

MINUTE 1 The windmill (p34)

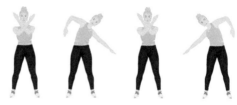

MINUTE 2 Standing waist bends (p44)

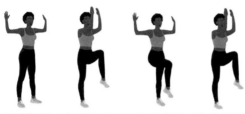

MINUTE 3 Marching arms (p52)

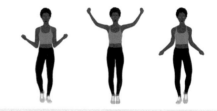

MINUTE 4 Skip to sculpt (p58)

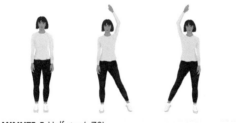

MINUTE 5 Half star (p70)

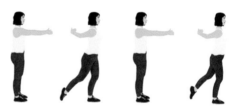

MINUTE 6 Shoulder sculpt & bottom lift (p124)

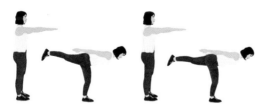

MINUTE 7 The glute doctor (p134)

WORKOUT 2: *If you spend all day on your feet*

Great if you want to give your feet a rest but give your body a workout!

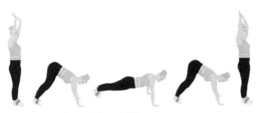

MINUTE 1 The walkdown (p38)

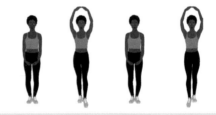

MINUTE 2 The ab makeover (p46)

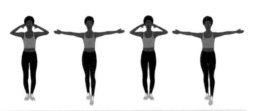

MINUTE 3 T-shirt tone arms (p60)

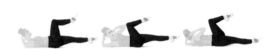

MINUTE 4 Ballerina arms (p62)

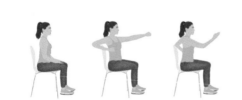

MINUTE 5 Run punch (p88)

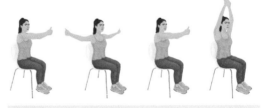

MINUTE 6 Thumbs up (p98)

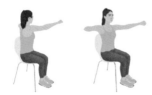

MINUTE 7 Cupid's arrow (p100)

WORKOUT 3: *If you are a new mother*

This workout is diastasis recti-friendly and will help repair any
abdominal separation, as well as strengthening your pelvic floor.

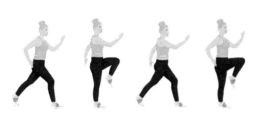

MINUTE 1 Sprinters' ab crunch (p42)

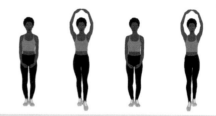

MINUTE 2 Ballerina arms (p62)

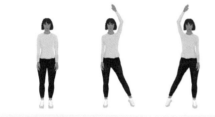

MINUTE 3 Half star (p70)

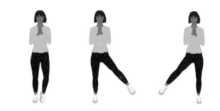

MINUTE 4 Ultimate thigh toner (p74)

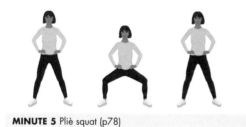

MINUTE 5 Plié squat (p78)

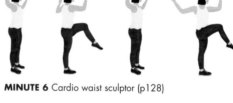

MINUTE 6 Cardio waist sculptor (p128)

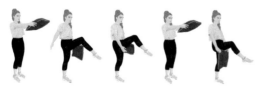

MINUTE 3 Under-knee pass (p146)

WORKOUT 4: *If you are recovering from injury*

These 7 moves will help rebuild core strength as well as working your major muscle groups, and all are low-impact, so ideal after an injury. (PS I hope you feel better soon.)

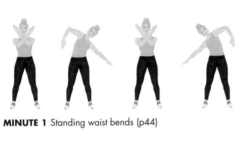

MINUTE 1 Standing waist bends (p44)

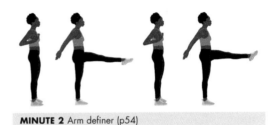

MINUTE 2 Arm definer (p54)

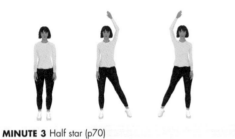

MINUTE 3 Half star (p70)

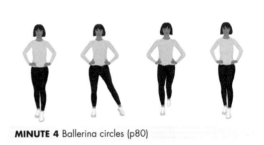

MINUTE 4 Ballerina circles (p80)

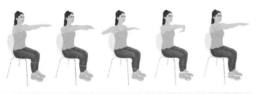

MINUTE 5 Sprint swim (p92)

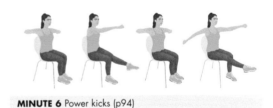

MINUTE 6 Power kicks (p94)

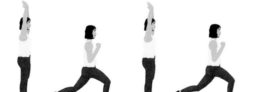
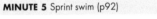

MINUTE 7 Lunge pull downs (p132)

WORKOUT 5: *If you are a runner*

A good set of exercises that will help increase your running speed and endurance.

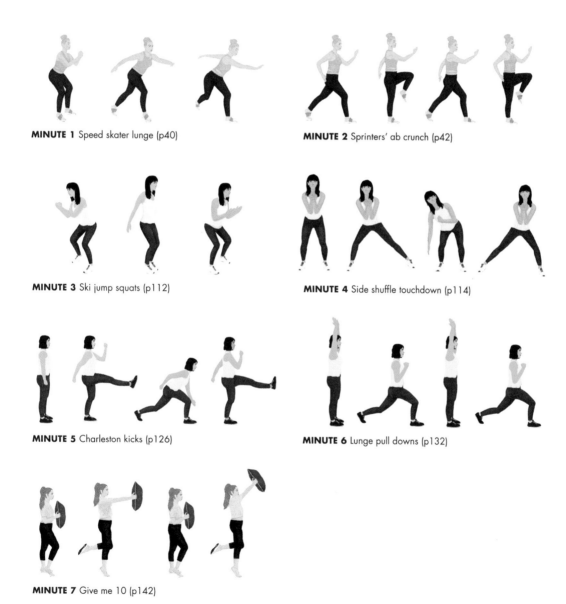

MINUTE 1 Speed skater lunge (p40)

MINUTE 2 Sprinters' ab crunch (p42)

MINUTE 3 Ski jump squats (p112)

MINUTE 4 Side shuffle touchdown (p114)

MINUTE 5 Charleston kicks (p126)

MINUTE 6 Lunge pull downs (p132)

MINUTE 7 Give me 10 (p142)

WORKOUT 6: *If you've fallen off the wagon*

7 great moves that are all feel-good exercises and are not taxing, so you can ease yourself back in slowly.

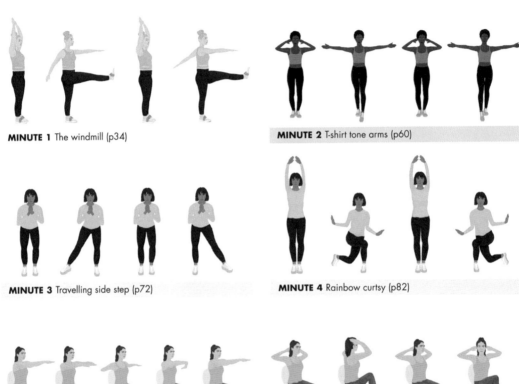

MINUTE 1 The windmill (p34)

MINUTE 2 T-shirt tone arms (p60)

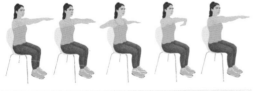

MINUTE 3 Travelling side step (p72)

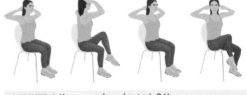

MINUTE 4 Rainbow curtsy (p82)

MINUTE 5 Sprint swim (p92)

MINUTE 6 Knee crunch and twist (p96)

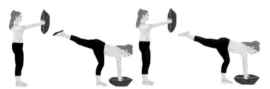

MINUTE 7 Touch down (p148)

WORKOUT 7: *If you're menopausal*

A workout that will help boost your natural metabolic rate back up, keep
your bones strong, and help reduce mood swings and hot flashes.

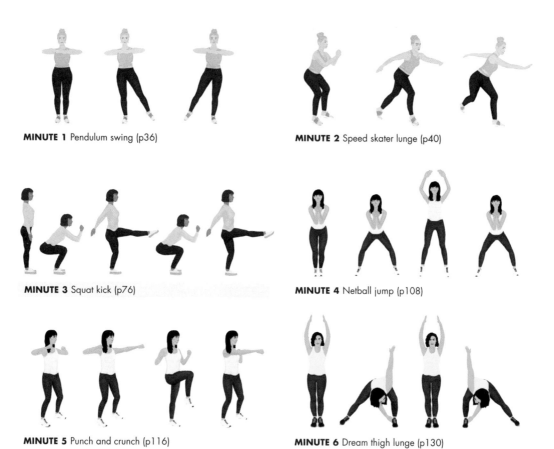

MINUTE 1 Pendulum swing (p36)

MINUTE 2 Speed skater lunge (p40)

MINUTE 3 Squat kick (p76)

MINUTE 4 Netball jump (p108)

MINUTE 5 Punch and crunch (p116)

MINUTE 6 Dream thigh lunge (p130)

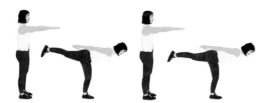

MINUTE 7 The glute doctor (p134)

LIFELONG FITNESS

7 TIPS

This chapter on maintaining the best version of you is the most important in the book. It's where I hand over to you, so you can maintain your own healthy lifestyle journey. Keeping going is vital.

All of us have the odd day when we struggle with motivation, even those of us who work in health and fitness. Here are 7 tips from me, that I often use myself, on how to turn that around and go from zero motivation to full-on ready-set-go!

1 THINK OF THE RESULTS YOU WANT.

Every personal goal you set yourself in life will need an investment from you. This totally applies to every aspect of your lives: you need to invest in your fitness, in your education and career, and especially in relationships. When you are struggling a little bit and telling yourself that you don't want to work out, or you don't need to exercise, or you're too busy to fit in 7 minutes, or too tired, say to yourself: I am going to give 100 per cent to this workout today and I will get 100 per cent back. We simply get out what we put in. Remember: you are doing this for you.

2 BE READY.

Have your 7-minute workout outfit always prepared, clean, and on hand, so you don't have to rummage around in drawers and cupboards to find your sports bra or leggings. Once dressed in your fitness gear, you are ready to work out, and on some days that can be half the battle! So be your own best friend and have it ready to jump into straight away.

3 REWARD YOURSELF FOR EACH 7-DAY CHALLENGE.

Say, for example, you are doing the 7-minute Dream arms workout (see p50): treat yourself to a lovely T-shirt to show off your toned arms. To "earn" the money to get that top, set yourself a fee for every time you complete your 7-minute arm workout. That fee goes in a savings jar. Come day 7, you'll have earned enough to get that T-shirt. For the Love my legs workout, this could be new shorts or new jeans; the LBD workout goes without saying… you get my drift.

4 YOU ARE FIT, DON'T FORGET IT.

And you may still have to convince your own mind of that! The fitter we are, the more likely we are to stay on the right road. It doesn't matter what age or ability you are, if you have done some form of exercise, consider yourself fit. You deserve that title; it's not just for sportspeople, but for everyone who is investing in their own health. Be excited to remember you are in the "fit gang" and use it to keep on track.

5 WHAT YOU DO TODAY WILL AFFECT YOUR FUTURE HEALTH.

Let that fact be a sharp but positive nudge to keep doing your exercises and eating well, as both your body and mind will look after you in return, now and in the years to come.

6 FOCUS ON HOW YOU'LL FEEL.

After your workout, you know you will feel exhilarated. When you have put in the effort, you will be completely energized for the day, and you can consider yourself a winner. So stay positive and remember to be so proud of yourself. Quite simply, you'll feel like a superwoman. That feeling is priceless

and – guess what – you will have it if you just do that 7-minute workout.

7 SET AN ALARM.

Every day, schedule in your workout, just as you would any other regular appointment. Do it now: set yourself an alert, or a reminder, on your phone. Add an inspirational ring tone, if you think it will help, perhaps your favourite workout song. When you make something a routine it becomes a habit, and that habit slots into your daily routine right back. Simply, it becomes part of your lifestyle.

Tip

We all have days when we're not really "feeling it" in terms of working out, due to hormones, tiredness, or life events. Don't let that stop you: do the workout anyway. If you don't perform as well as usual, just chalk it up to experience, try again next time, and remember: you're still lapping the old version of you that used to spend that 7 minutes just lying on the couch.

INDEX

ACKNOWLEDGEMENTS

To be able to work with Dorling Kindersley and bring to life my 7-minute workouts in book form is a dream come true, and watching it unfold has been one of my biggest "Yes I Can" moments!

But this has not been done alone, and I have so many people to thank. First is my family, and especially my Mum and Dad, who taught me to work hard and be someone who gives in life. Their values have been the making of me. I am so lucky to have such a close, supportive, and loving family who help me so much in so many ways.

I would like to thank Jody for making this happen, and Mary-Clare for having the dream team that have helped create a book that I am so proud of. And, of course, a special big thank you to both Michaels, and to Anna, Hatti, and Ellie.

Most importantly, thank you to every single one of my followers. You have all been with me on this adventure. I'm so grateful. #Lucyssquad is growing daily, as we are becoming our best, and supporting each other along the way.

PUBLISHER'S ACKNOWLEDGEMENTS

Author photographer Ruth Jenkinson
Author food styling Jane Lawrie
Author hair and make-up Jo McKenna
Recipe photography food styling Kate Wesson
Recipe photography art direction Sara Robin
Recipe photography prop styling Rob Merrett
Image retouching Steve Crozier
Proofreader Kathy Steer
Indexer Vanessa Bird

The information in this book has been compiled as general guidance on the specific subjects addressed. It is not a substitute and not to be relied on for medical, healthcare, or pharmaceutical professional advice. Please consult your GP before changing, stopping, or starting any medical treatment. So far as the author is aware the information given is correct and up to date as at October 2019. Practice, laws, and regulations all change and the reader should obtain up to date professional advice on any such issues. All weight-loss stories and photographs have been supplied independently by members of the public and have not been verified by the author or the publishers. The author and publishers disclaim, as far as the law allows, any liability arising directly or indirectly from the use or misuse of the information contained in this book.

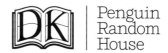

DK UK
Editors Lucy Bannell, Amy Slack
Designer Hannah Moore
Editorial Assistant Millie Andrew
Illustrator Sophie State
Jacket designer Amy Cox
Jackets co-ordinator Lucy Philpott
Producer, pre-production David Almond
Senior producer Stephanie McConnell
Managing editor Stephanie Farrow
Managing art editor Christine Keilty
Art director Maxine Pedliham
Publisher Mary-Clare Jerram

This edition published in 2019
First published in Great Britain in 2019 by
Dorling Kindersley Limited
80 Strand, London, WC2R 0RL

A CIP catalogue record for this book
is available from the British Library.
ISBN: 978-0-2414-3003-3

Printed and bound in Slovakia

A WORLD OF IDEAS:
SEE ALL THERE IS TO KNOW

www.dk.com

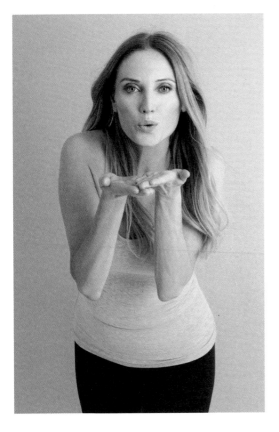

ABOUT LUCY

Lucy Wyndham-Read has helped (literally) 100,000s of people worldwide to successfully reach their health goals, from better fitness and nutrition to weight loss.

Her unique 7-minute home workout method of training is a truly global phenomenon, with more than 1 million subscribers to her YouTube channel and an incredible 44 million views for her "7 Day Challenge" video (which places it among the most-liked fitness videos ever shared on the platform). Lucy has more than 1.5 million followers across social media, and has created one of the fastest-growing online communities dedicated to fitness, health, and wellbeing.

Lucy has more than 20 years' experience in fitness, healthy living, and motivation. She appears frequently on television, including Sky News, BBC1, Channel 4, and Channel 5. Her workouts have been featured by the media worldwide, and even doctors have prescribed them to their patients.

Lucy's mission has always been to educate and to show people how to get results. She truly believes she can help everyone look and feel their best. Her followers have achieved amazing results, and Lucy's message of self-confidence and self-respect helps them to reach their goals with the correct mindset and the right fitness plan. Lucy, and her followers, live by the phrase "Yes I Can".

Find me on:

Instagram @LucyWyndhamRead
Twitter @LucyWyndhamRead
Facebook LucysSquad

Post your 7-minute workout pictures, or photos of recipes from the book, and tag me. You can also use the hashtag #7minutebodyplan. I can't wait to see how you are getting on!